The American Civil War Surgery Series

Edited by Ira M. Rutkow, M.D., Dr.P.H.

1. S.D. Gross: *A Manual of Military Surgery* (Philadelphia, 1861)
2. S.P. Moore: *A Manual of Military Surgery, Prepared for the Use of the Confederate States Army* (Richmond, 1863)
3. S.W. Mitchell, G.R. Morehouse and W.W. Keen: *Gunshot Wounds and Other Injuries of Nerves* (Philadelphia, 1864)
4. J.J. Chisolm: *A Manual of Military Surgery* (Richmond, 1861)
5. F.H. Hamilton: *A Practical Treatise on Military Surgery* (New York, 1861)
6. E. Warren: *An Epitome of Practical Surgery for Field and Hospital* (Richmond, 1863)
7. C.S. Tripler and G.C. Blackman: *Hand-book for the Military Surgeon* (Cincinnati, 1861)
8. S. Smith: *Hand-book of Surgical Operations* (New York, 1862)
9. F. Formento: *Notes and Observations on Army Surgery* (New Orleans, 1863), bound with:

   M. Schuppert: *A Treatise on Gun-shot Wounds: Written for and Dedicated to the Surgeons of the Confederate States Army* (New Orleans, 1861)
10. J.H. Packard: *A Manual of Minor Surgery* (Philadelphia, 1863)
11. Adjutant-General and the Surgeon-General: *List of Battles and Roster of Regimental Surgeons and Assistant Surgeons During the War of the Rebellion* (Washington, D.C., 1883)

HAND-BOOK FOR THE MILITARY SURGEON

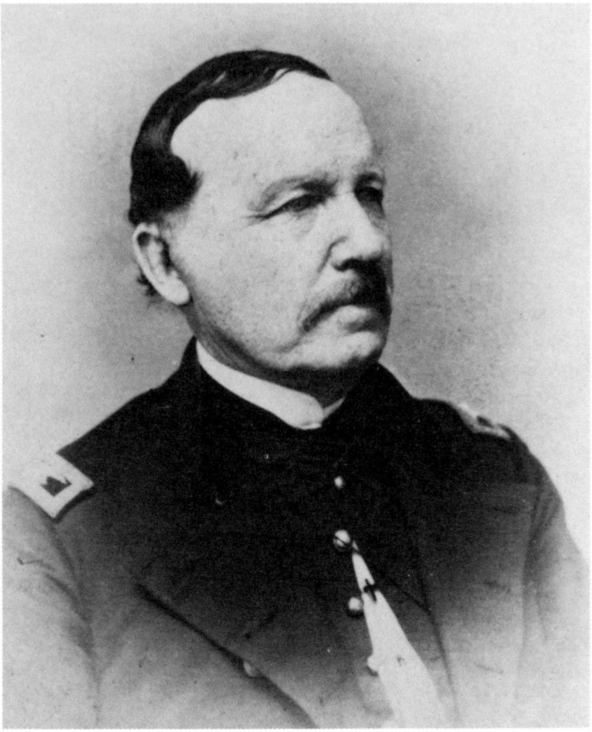

Charles Stuart Tripler

1806–1866

National Library of Medicine

HAND-BOOK FOR THE MILITARY SURGEON

by
Charles Stuart Tripler, M.D.
and
George Curtis Blackman, M.D.

Reprinted with a Biographical Introduction

by Ira M. Rutkow, M.D., Dr.P.H.

Norman Publishing
San Francisco
1989

Published by Norman Publishing
Division of Jeremy Norman & Co., Inc.
442 Post Street
San Francisco, California 94102–1579

Library of Congress Cataloging-in-Publication Data

Tripler, Chas. S. (Charles Stuart), 1806–1866.
Handbook for the military surgeon.

(American Civil War surgery series ; 7)
Reprint. Originally published: Hand-book for the military surgeon. Cincinnati : R. Clarke, 1861.
1. Surgery, Military—Handbooks, manuals, etc.
I. Blackman, George Curtis, 1819–1871. II. Title. III. Title: Hand-book for the military surgeon. IV. Series: American Civil War surgery series ; no. 7.
[DNLM: WO T835h 1861a]
RD153.T75 1989 617'.99 88–60672
ISBN 0–930405–06–4

The American Civil War Surgery Series, No. 7

This is a reproduction of the first edition, printed in Cincinnati in 1861. Irregularities in the printing appear exactly as they do in the original edition.

This book is printed on acid-free paper, and its binding materials have been chosen for strength and durability.

Manufactured in the United States of America.

Charles Stuart Tripler

Charles Stuart Tripler was born in New York's Bowery on January 19, 1806. His mother was the daughter of a former governor of Bermuda. Because of reverses in his father's business, Tripler was apprenticed while still a youngster to Stephen Brown, an apothecary who was also a graduate in medicine. Tripler obtained most of his secondary education through this arrangement, with Brown instructing him after business hours. Because of Brown's medical orientation, Tripler decided to matriculate at the College of Physicians and Surgeons in New York, from which he graduated in 1827.

After graduation Tripler served for a while as resident physician at Bellevue Hospital. During this time, he contracted a mild case of smallpox. With his formal medical training at an end, Tripler moved to West Point with the idea of entering the army medical service. There he assisted Walter V. Wheaton (1787–1860) in his duties as post surgeon and in some private practice. Tripler was well liked by many of the officers, and was allowed to take courses in mathematics and languages with the cadet corps. He finally obtained permission to take the examination for the medical service and was commissioned as an assistant surgeon in October 1830.

Tripler's first two assignments took him to Maine and Louisiana. In the winter of 1836, he was transferred to Florida, where for three years he took part in field duty against the Seminole Indians. In July 1838, Tripler was promoted to full surgeon, and in 1839 was reassigned to Buffalo. The following January, he was sent to Detroit.

In May 1846, the Mexican War broke out, and Tripler was made medical director of a division of regular troops. Although Tripler was commended in numerous reports, he was very critical of the soldiers, especially of what he regarded as their inferior physical stamina. He thought this weakness was a direct cause of the fevers, diarrheas, and dysentery which many soldiers contracted.

Following the capture of Mexico City, Tripler was given the task of organizing and operating a general hospital for the army by the newly appointed medical director, Richard Satterlee (1798–1880). He remained in Mexico City until April 1848, when he and another surgeon, Presley H. Craig (?–1848), were placed in charge of patients in Jalapa following the armistice. Tripler returned to his post at Detroit shortly thereafter and served through 1852. In 1849, he was elected president of the fledgling Michigan State Medical Society.

In May 1850, Tripler was sent as a delegate by the Medical Society to the third annual meeting of the American Medical Association in Cincinnati. Surgeon-General Thomas Lawson (1795–1861) took advantage of his presence to appoint him to represent the Medical Department of the Army at the meeting. This was the first occasion at which representatives of the army attended a meeting of the national society. At that time, the government first proposed the conferring of military rank on medical officers in the army. Tripler later served as vice-president of the American Medical Association.

In June 1852, Tripler was ordered to New York to accompany troops to the West Coast by way of Panama. He remained in California for four years, building up a flourishing private practice in general medicine. Returning to the East via Panama, Tripler assumed a post in April 1856 in Kentucky just a few miles from Cincinnati. This barracks became the major recruiting depot for the western half of the United States.

While stationed in Kentucky, Tripler prepared a major work, the *Manual of the Medical Officer of the Army of the United States: Part 1, Recruiting and the Inspection of Recruits* (1858). This book was to be part of a projected series, but the other volumes were never completed. Upon its publication, the work became accepted throughout the army as the ultimate authority on recruitment standards. A second edition was printed in 1866, and an epitome of it was prepared in 1884.

Soon after settling in Kentucky, Tripler associated himself with the Medical College of Ohio in Cincinnati. He also published some minor papers on delirium tremens and medical delusions. In the winter of 1860–61, he prepared a course of lectures on military surgery in conjunction with George Blackman (1819–1871), who was professor of surgery at the same school. Out of these lectures came the *Hand-book for the Military Surgeon* (1861). A second edition was printed the same year. However, this book met with much less success than his previous work.

With the start of the Civil War, Tripler was assigned to Washington and appointed medical director of the Army of the Shenandoah. When General George McClellan (1826–1885) assumed command of the Army of the Potomac, Tripler became its general director (August 1861). He soon set about organizing the army's general medical services, including consideration of plans to establish field hospitals and an ambulance service. However, to his discredit he did not follow through on efforts toward organizing the ambulance corps and only half-heartedly supported the concept of field hospitals.

The Peninsula Campaign began in April 1862, and resulted in large numbers of casualties. Indirectly, this indecisive battle brought tremendous discredit to the medical service and to Tripler. Strong criticism was directed at the army's health services by the United States Sanitary Commission, a powerful civilian organization involved in the medical direction of the war effort. Jonathan Letterman (1824–1872) was sent to relieve Tripler, who was offered his choice of stations for reassignment. He decided to return to Detroit, but soon moved to Columbus and still later to Cincinnati, where he served until the end of the war.

Tripler's reputation suffered as a result of his failures during the Peninsula Campaign; however, up to that time he had enjoyed a brilliant career in the army's medical department. Unfortunately, he lacked the overall vision that Letterman brought to the task. Nevertheless, he was a talented physician and an excellent surgeon. President Lincoln (1809–1865) nominated

Tripler as Inspector-General, but the nomination was never confirmed by Congress.

Tripler married Eunice Hunt in 1841, and they had several children. In her eighty-ninth year, while living in Nebraska, she published her memoirs entitled *Eunice Tripler: Some Notes of Her Personal Recollections* (1910).

In 1860, Columbia University conferred upon Tripler the honorary degree of M.A. For about three years before his death, he was the medical director of the Department of the Ohio. He was given the brevet of colonel in November 1864, and that of brigadier general in March 1865. While serving in Cincinnati in early 1866, he developed a highly invasive squamous cell carcinoma of the head and neck, which resulted in his death on October 20. Interment was in the Elmwood Cemetery in Detroit.

Tripler is remembered today chiefly for his *Manual*, which for half a century was the standard guide for all army recruit examiners. His name is also memorialized by the Tripler General Hospital in Honolulu.

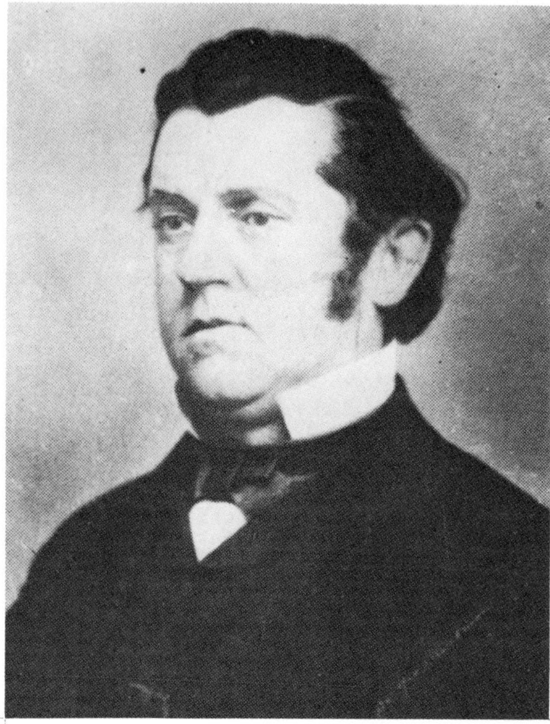

George Curtis Blackman
1819–1871

Courtesy of the New York Academy of Medicine Library

George Curtis Blackman

Born in Bridgeport, Connecticut, on April 21, 1819, George Curtis Blackman was the son of Thomas Blackman, a judge from Newton, Connecticut. He obtained most of his early education in Bridgeport and in Newburgh, New York. Blackman received his undergraduate education at Yale University and studied medicine at the College of Physicians and Surgeons in New York City, from which he graduated in March 1840. He immediately began to practice in various dispensaries in New York, but severe tuberculosis marked by repeated hemorrhages forced him to close his practice.

On the advice of friends who suggested that he take sea air as a cure, Blackman decided to pursue further studies in Europe. To finance these plans, he took a position as surgeon on various Atlantic packet ships, allegedly crossing the ocean thirty-six times. He was able to spend considerable time in London and Paris as a result of this work, and in 1845 became an occasional student at the London Hospital.

Blackman's studies in London were hampered by his lack of money—so much so that he is said to have subsisted on two penny rolls a day, and to have kept himself warm with only his blankets to avoid the expense of a fire. Blackman later became one of the very few foreign surgeons elected to the Royal Medical and Chirurgical Society.

In the late 1840s, with much improved health and a European medical education, Blackman worked his way back to the United States on a Liverpool vessel as assistant surgeon. He resettled in Newburgh, New York, where he practiced for a number of years. During this period, he wrote numerous essays and reviews for medical journals. Among his most outstanding accomplishments was his translation from the French of Auguste Vidal's (1803–1856) *Traité des maladies vénériennes* (1853).

In 1854, Blackman was chosen professor of surgery at the Medical College of Ohio in Cincinnati on the recommendation of some of the most eminent surgeons in America. There he established a reputation as a superb technical surgeon and outstanding clinical teacher. Valentine Mott (1785–1865), who considered Blackman an expert in the literature of surgery, asked him to edit his previous translation of the three-volume *New Elements of Operative Surgery* by Alfred Velpeau (1795–

1867). Blackman completed this enormous task in 1856 after having made numerous additions and emendations. While in Cincinnati, Blackman also served as an associate editor of the *Western Lancet* and the *Cincinnati Journal of Medicine*, and for many years was a frequent contributor to various medical journals. In addition, he practiced at several Cincinnati hospitals, including Commercial Hospital, Good Samaritan, St. Mary's, and St. John's.

In October 1861, Blackman was appointed a brigade surgeon of volunteers to the United States Army and was in field service in the South as medical director to the Army of the Cumberland. While in this capacity, he saw action at the Battle of Shiloh. Later he was transferred to the staff of General George McClellan (1826–1885) and was present at the Battle of the Wilderness. He also served for a short time on the Ohio State Medical Board for the army.

Aside from his *Hand-book for the Military Surgeon*, Blackman did not author any other books. At the time of his death, he was working on a textbook concerning the principles and practice of surgery and on a treatise to be titled *Legal Liability in Surgical Malpractice*; neither was ever published.

Blackman was reputed to have been quite temperamental. Although he had a rather large clinical practice, he was such a poor manager that he died destitute. Samuel David Gross (1805–1884) speculated in his autobiography that Blackman was addicted to opium during the later years of his life. Whether this could have contributed to his early demise is unknown, although Blackman died of liver failure after being ill for only a few weeks.

In 1855, Blackman married Agnes Addington of New York. Together they had two sons and a daughter. He died in his home in Avondale, Ohio, on July 19, 1871. Interment was in the Spring Grove Cemetery of that town.

HAND-BOOK

FOR THE

MILITARY SURGEON:

BEING A COMPENDIUM OF

THE DUTIES OF THE MEDICAL OFFICER IN THE FIELD, THE SANITARY MANAGEMENT OF THE CAMP, THE PREPARATION OF FOOD, ETC.; WITH FORMS FOR THE REQUISITIONS FOR SUPPLIES, RETURNS, ETC.; THE DIAGNOSIS AND TREATMENT OF CAMP DYSENTERY; AND ALL THE IMPORTANT POINTS IN

WAR SURGERY:

INCLUDING GUNSHOT WOUNDS, AMPUTATION, WOUNDS OF THE CHEST, ABDOMEN, ARTERIES AND HEAD, AND THE USE OF CHLOROFORM.

BY

CHAS. S. TRIPLER, A.M., M.D.,
Surgeon United States Army.

AND

GEORGE C. BLACKMAN, M.D.,
Professor of Surgery in the Medical College of Ohio, Surgeon to the Commercial Hospital, St. John's Hospital, etc.

CINCINNATI:
ROBERT CLARKE & CO., PUBLISHERS,
No. 55 West Fourth Street.
1861.

E. MORGAN & SONS,
Stereotypers, Printers and Binders,
111 MAIN STREET.

PREFACE.

The want of a work like the present is seriously felt by those now about to engage for the first time in the duties of Military Surgery. To supply this want, the publishers requested Dr. CHAS. S. TRIPLER, U. S. A., to consent to the issue of the lectures which for the last three years he has delivered in the Medical College of Ohio, by invitation of the Professor of Surgery in that institution. To this the Doctor kindly consented. The publishers likewise requested Professor BLACKMAN to supply the material for the chapters on Wounds of the Abdomen, Head, and Arteries—which he has attempted, after very brief notice, amid most pressing engagements. Prof. B. wishes it to be distinctly understood that his only aim has been to compile from the best sources within his reach such a digest as will promote the objects proposed by the publishers.

In addition to his own task, Prof. B. has been compelled to arrange three of the lectures of Dr. TRIPLER from unfinished notes, left with him by Dr. T., who was summoned to report himself to headquarters before his revision of his labors was completed. This, it is hoped, will be a sufficient apology for any imperfections which may be detected. A chapter on the Use of Chloroform has been added, taken from the valuable work of Mr. Macleod on the Crimean War, which will be found of interest.

CINCINNATI, MAY 10, 1861.

CONTENTS.

CONTENTS OF APPENDIX.

HAND-BOOK

FOR

THE MILITARY SURGEON.

CHAPTER I.

DUTIES OF THE MEDICAL OFFICER.—ORGANIZATION OF FIELD HOSPITALS.—MODES OF PROCURING SUPPLIES.

THE military medical officer is charged with the whole sanitary care of his corps. He is not to suppose that he is to sit in his tent, and when called upon to see a patient, he is to repair to the bedside of the sick, prescribe and retire, as in civil life. On the contrary, he is most valuable when having carefully reflected upon the laws of Hygiene, so that he has them at his fingers' ends, he is ready to apply them to the emergency before him, so as to afford to the troops under his immediate charge, the greatest possible security against the invasion of disease. Nothing so much embarrasses operations in a campaign, as a large sick report. Upon marches, the sick require transportation and nursing. Every nurse is an effective man lost to the fighting force. Every wagon employed in the hospital department, is so much lost to the supply train of the army. To limit this loss as much as possible, should be the constant effort of the zealous medical officer.

But however scientific, zealous, intelligent and active the medical officer may be, men *will* get sick, and in a fight, they *will* get wounded. The sick and wounded must be cared for. They must have hospitals, medicines, instruments, hospital stores, bedding, and the like. The inexperienced medical officer can not provide these without knowing, from some source, what he wants, and where he is to get it. I shall therefore, in the first place, endeavor to give him this information.

Medicines, instruments, dressings, hospital stores, and bedding, are furnished by the medical purveyor, upon requisitions made by the senior surgeon of a regiment, or separate commands. In the field, these requisitions are to be approved by the medical director. If there is no medical director present, a special requisition may be approved by the commanding officer; and if there be no medical purveyor within reach, the supplies may be purchased by the quartermaster.

These supplies in the army, are required to be made according to the standard supply table; and if any article is not in accordance with that table, the reason therefor must be set forth on the requisition. Forms for these requisitions, accounts for articles purchased, etc., are appended to this book.

The senior medical officer of a division or separate corps d'armee, is ex officio, the medical director. A medical officer should be detailed by the medical director, to act as medical purveyor. There should be at the depots for the supplies, a medical purveyor in charge of all those pertaining to the hospital department. This officer is expected to be always in condition to supply such requisitions as may be made upon him by the medical officers in the field.

The quartermaster's department provides "the quarters and transportation of the army, storage and transportation for all army supplies, army clothing, camp and garrison equipage, cavalry and artillery horses, fuel, forage, straw and stationery." *

"Estimates of the medical director, approved by the commanding officer, for the necessary transportation to be provided for the hospital service, will be furnished to the quartermaster."

"The sick will be transported on the application of the medical officers."

"The allowance and change of straw for the sick, is regulated by the surgeon." *

Tents and camp equipage are furnished by the quartermaster's department.

The allowance for a surgeon in the field, is two tents, one ax, one hatchet; for an assistant surgeon, one tent, one ax, one hatchet.

These are for the personal use of these officers, and they are required to render quarterly returns of them to the quartermaster general.

---

* Army regulations, Art. 41.

Requisitions for all these articles are to be made upon the quartermaster's department.

Medical officers receive their stationery from the medical purveyor and not from the quartermaster.

When men are sick in hospital, returns for their subsistence are to be made to the commissary of subsistence, by the senior medical officer, at such stated periods as may be determined by the commanding officer. The Form for this return will be found in the appendix.

Issues to the hospital will be on returns by the medical officer, for such provisions only as are actually required for the sick and the attendants. The cost of such parts of the ration as are issued, will be charged to the hospital at contract or cost prices, and the hospital will be credited by the whole number of complete rations due through the month, at contract or cost prices; the balance, constituting the hospital fund, or any portion of it, may be expended by the commissary, on the requisition of the medical officer, in the purchase of any article for the subsistence or comfort of the sick, not authorized to be otherwise furnished.*

"The ration is three fourths of a pound of pork or bacon, or one and a fourth pounds of fresh or salt beef; eighteen ounces of bread or flour, or twelve ounces of hard bread, or one and a fourth pounds corn meal; and at the rate, to one hundred rations, of eight quarts of peas or beans, or, in lieu thereof, ten pounds of rice ; ten pounds of coffee; fifteen pounds of sugar; four quarts of vinegar, one and a half pounds of tallow, or one and a fourth pounds of adamantine or one pound of sperm candles; four pounds of soap, and two quarts of salt."

"On a campaign, or on marches, or on board of transports, the ration of hard bread is one pound."

The medical officer determines how much of each of these articles he will require for the subsistence of the sick in his hospital during the period for which the return is made. With the fund accruing from the articles saved, he is authorized to call upon the commissary of subsistence, to purchase such comforts for the sick, as can be procured; such as milk, butter, eggs, chickens, fresh vegetables, and the like. With careful and judicious management, the savings of the rations are always sufficient for this purpose.

Tea, arrow-root, farina, nutmegs, brandy and whiskey, are sup-

---

* Army regulations, Art. 42.

plied by the medical purveyor. The medical officer selects the cooks, nurses and matrons for his hospital. These selections must be approved by the commanding officer. The cooks and nurses are taken from the privates of the regiment. They are exempted from all other duty, except the parades for muster, and the weekly inspection of their companies. When their services are necessary with the sick, they are also excused from these, by the commanding officer, upon the application of the surgeon. The allowance of hospital attendants for troops in the field, is, for one company, one steward, one nurse and one cook; for each additional company, one nurse; and for commands of over five companies, one additional cook. The duties of the steward are, to take charge of the medicines, hospital stores and supplies; to put up the prescriptions of the medical officer; to see to their distribution and administration to the sick; to enter in a book, daily, the issues to the cooks and nurses; to prepare the provision returns, and receive and distribute the rations. The cooks and nurses are under his orders; he is responsible for the cleanliness of the wards, tents and kitchens, patients and attendants, and all articles in use. He will ascertain who are present at sunrise, at sunset, and at tattoo, and report absentees.

These duties are too important to be entrusted entirely to the steward; they must be constantly superintended by the surgeon and his assistants. Frequent visits should be made to the hospital by the surgeon, and he should require each of his assistants to be responsible for their exact performance in his turn.

In camp, an hour is always fixed by the commanding officer, for each particular duty. At the proper time, the surgeon's call is beaten. This is usually a quarter of an hour before, or a quarter of an hour after breakfast. In my opinion, it is better that it should be beaten after breakfast.

"At the surgeon's call, the sick, then in the companies, will be conducted to the hospital by the first sergeants, who will each hand to the surgeon, in his company book, a list of all the sick of the company, on which the surgeon shall state who are to remain or go into hospital; who are to return to quarters, as sick or convalescent; what duties the convalescents in quarters are capable of; what cases are feigned; and any other information he may have to communicate to the company commander." *

---

* Regulations of medical department U. S. Army.

"Patients in hospital are, if possible, to leave their arms and accouterments with their companies, and in no case to take ammunition into the hospital." *

Upon marches, the surgeon's call is usually sounded as soon as the hospital tent, appropriated to the supplies, is pitched and arranged, at the close of the day's march. At the surgeon's call, a medical officer, to be designated by the surgeon, repairs promptly to the hospital tent, to examine and prescribe for the sick. When there are many sick, all the medical officers should attend the surgeon's call.

Immediately after the examination of the sick, the morning report of the surgeon is made out and sent to the adjutant's office, for the information of the commanding officer. This report is always signed by the senior medical officer, and he is responsible that it is correct. The Form for this report is in the appendix.

In the field, the senior medical officer of a regiment, or separate command, must keep a register of patients, a prescription and diet book, a case-book, and order, and letter-book. The army Forms for these books are appended.

When troops are ordered to move, there will usually be found, in the hospital, some patients too ill to accompany their regiment. General hospitals are established at some convenient points, for the reception of these patients. When men are sent to a general hospital, it is the duty of the captain of the company to which they belong, to send accurate descriptive lists of the men with them. Where this duty is neglected, it is impossible for the surgeon, in charge of the general hospital, to muster them for payment, to take proper care of their clothing, arms, and other effects, or to inform their captains of the result of their cases.

Sometimes, upon a march, a man becomes too ill to bear further transportation, and it is necessary to leave him in a private hospital, or private house. The descriptive list should then be left with him, in the care of the person taking charge of the man. It is incumbent upon the medical officer, to urge upon the captains the strict fulfillment of this duty. Every consideration of policy and humanity requires it should be done.

When a patient is sent to a general hospital, it is the duty of the medical officer to send with him, to the surgeon of the hospital, a

---

* Regulations of medical department U. S. Army.

report containing the history of his case, with the treatment up to that time. This duty must never be neglected. Men are frequently received into the general hospitals, too ill to give any account of themselves; their *lives* may be the penalty of the neglect of their own surgeons, in failing to comply with this simple requirement.

The senior medical officer is required to make the muster and pay rolls of the steward, matrons, cooks, and nurses, attached to his hospital, on the forms furnished from the adjutant-general's office.

The pay of the steward, is that of the orderly sergeant of a company, of a matron, six dollars per month and one ration per day. The cooks and nurses are allowed twenty-five cents per day, extra pay. It is the last item only, that is entered upon the hospital rolls—the men are mustered upon their company rolls for their regular pay.

The senior medical officer is required to make, "monthly, to the medical director, and quarterly, to the surgeon general, a report of sick and wounded, and of deaths, and of certificates for discharge for disability." * The Form is in the appendix.

Medical officers in charge of medical supplies, make returns of them annually, on the 31st December, or whenever they are relieved from the charge of them, to the surgeon general. When these supplies are turned over to another officer, the officer delivering them must hand duplicate invoices of them to his successor, or take from him duplicate receipts. He sends one copy of these receipts to the surgeon general with his returns. The Form for these returns is appended.

Fuel for the use of the hospital is to be furnished by the quartermaster upon the return of the surgeon, countersigned by the commanding officer. Straw for filling the bedsacks is furnished by the quartermaster upon the requisition of the surgeon. It takes 12 or 14 pounds of straw for each bedsack.

It is not contemplated to use bedsacks in the field, in the army service. They can not be carried upon a march. But in permanent camps, they may be necessary. In that case, the maximum number required will be 80 for 1,000 men. A supply table for field service has been carefully prepared by a board of army surgeons. It will be found in the appendix. It will show at once to the inexperienced surgeon what he wants for commands of any size for a period of

---

* Regulations of medical department U. S. Army.

three months. If he can procure his supplies from an army medical purveyor, it will only be necessary for him to state the strength of the command, and the time for which the supplies are required, and the proper quantity of each article will be furnished.

The number of tents that will probably be required for the hospital department, has been carefully estimated by an army medical board, and is as follows:

	HOSPITAL TENTS.	SIBLEY TENTS.	COMMON TENTS.
One company, - - - - - - -		1	1
Three companies, - - - - - -	1	1	1
Five companies, - - - - - -	2	1	1
Seven companies, - - - - - -	2	1	1
Ten companies, - - - - - -	3	1	1

The dimensions of the hospital tent referred to, are these: In length, 14 feet; in width, 15 feet; in hight (center), 11 feet; with a wall 4½ feet, and a fly of appropriate size.

Such a tent will accommodate 8 to 10 patients comfortably.

If tents of this pattern can not be furnished by the regimental quartermaster, the ordinary wall tent may be substituted. These tents are for the accommodation of the sick; the sibley and common tents, for the medical supplies, books, and nurses. The same board recommended "the adoption of a hospital knapsack, to be carried by a hospital orderly upon the march or in battle, who is habitually to follow the medical officer. The knapsack is to be made of light wood, to be divided into four compartments or drawers, and to be covered with canvas. The purpose of this knapsack is to carry, in an accessible shape, such instruments, dressings, and medicines as may be needed in an emergency on the march or in the field. The dimensions of the hospital knapsack to be those of the ordinary knapsack."

It will be at once perceived how convenient, and even necessary, such an arrangement is. Every medical officer should have one. An ambulance system for the army was recommended by the board, and adopted by the war department. A very few of these carriages have been made for trial, and so far as heard from, the results have been satisfactory. It is to be regretted that there is not in store a full supply for the present emergency.

The calculation upon which the system is based, is that four per cent. of the force will require transportation; one half of whom will be lying down.

With the new ambulances, a regiment is estimated to require two four-wheeled and ten two-wheeled ambulances; and in addition four two-wheeled transport carts—the latter for the hospital supplies, tents, cooking utensils, etc.

Under present circumstances, we are obliged to use the ordinary baggage wagon for our supplies and camp equipage. One wagon is sufficient for that purpose for a regiment, and as much as can be afforded. For the conveyance of the sick, we have to use such wagons of the train as are emptied or lightened of their loads by the the issue of supplies to the troops. The sick must be distributed among them to the best advantage. All that a medical officer can do in this emergency, is to report to the quartermaster that such a man requires transportation. It is the duty of the latter to provide it. Upon the march, the habitual place of the medical officer is at the rear of the regiment. A man who is taken sick, falls out from the ranks, and meets the surgeon as he comes up. He is then examined, prescribed for, and sent to the wagons or remanded to his company, as his case may require. If he is sent to the wagons, he should be furnished with a written permit for that privilege. Medical officers should be very careful in scrutinizing all such cases, or they will find the baggage train seriously embarrassed, and overloaded by men who are able enough to march.

In order to prevent the accumulation of stragglers at the rear, under pretext of seeing the surgeon, it is advisable for one of the medical officers to ride occasionally to the head of the column, and permit it to pass him on the march. Any man feeling ill, can then see him, and have his case decided on, without the necessity of falling behind his company. When a medical officer makes this movement, he should be careful always to pass to *leeward* of the column, that the dust he raises may be carried away from the men.

The following extracts from the General Regulations for the Army, will indicate the proper arrangements for the medical officers in battle:

"Before the action, the quartermaster of the division makes all the necessary arrangements for the transportation of the wounded. He establishes the ambulance depots in the rear, and gives his assistants the necessary instruction for the service of the ambulance wagons, and other means of removing the wounded."

"The ambulance depot to which the wounded are carried or directed for immediate treatment, is generally established at the most convenient building nearest the field of battle. A *red flag* marks its place or the way to it, to the conductors of the ambulances, and to the wounded who can walk."

"The active ambulances follow the troops engaged, to succor the wounded and remove them to the depots. For this purpose, the conductors should always have the necessary assistants, that the soldiers may have no excuse to leave the ranks for that purpose."

"The medical director of the division, after consultation with the quartermaster general, distributes the medical officers and hospital attendants at his disposal, to the depots and active ambulances. He will send officers and attendants, when practicable, to the active ambulances, to relieve the wounded who require treatment before being removed from the ground. He will see that the depots and ambulances are provided with the necessary apparatus, medicines and stores. He will take post and render his professional services at the principal depot."

"If the enemy endanger the depot, the quartermaster takes the orders of the general to remove it or to strengthen its guard."

"The wounded in the depots and the sick are removed, as soon as possible, to the hospitals that have been established by the quartermaster general of the army on the flanks or rear of the army."

This, I think, includes everything the inexperienced medical officer will feel at a loss about, in entering upon his duties with troops in campaign. If anything important is omitted, the haste with which the work is prepared must be my apology.

CHAPTER II.

MILITARY HYGIENE—PRESERVATION OF HEALTH OF TROOPS IN CAMPAIGN.

To the neglect of plain hygienic principles, I am persuaded, is to be attributed the greater portion of the diseases that scourge so constantly all armies in the field. Pure air; good and sufficient clothing; good, sufficient, and well-cooked food; temperance and cleanliness, are the important points. Soldiers in campaign will always have exercise enough.

In the army, these hygienic principles are always more or less observed; they form the basis of the regulations in relation to the police of barracks, camps, etc., the clothing and cooking of the men. In the volunteer service, they are not at all, or only imperfectly, observed, simply because they are not understood by either officers or men. Their importance is not appreciated, and the consequence is a marked disparity between the two descriptions of force in their losses by disease and death. Thus, in the war with Mexico, the relative losses of the volunteers and regulars of the old army from disease, was a 4.7 to 1; the deaths, 6.3 to 4.7. Excess of loss to volunteers, 50 per cent. There is no necessity whatever for this. It is due simply to ignorance of the laws of health on the one hand, and the constant observance of them on the other.

The first cause I shall notice in this connection, is the ordinary defects of the volunteer recruits. In the volunteers, almost all who offer are received. Thus, men debilitated by malarial cachexia, particularly at the West—by intemperance, etc., are generally received into the ranks. They look very well, and, so far as they can judge, they are very well; but, exposed to the fatigues and labors of the camp, they are almost sure to become sick.

In the regular army, on the other hand, every recruit is subjected to a rigorous inspection before he is received. He is examined, stripped, and every ordinary disqualification carefully inquired into. The result of this system was, that in 1852, of all applicants for enlistment, there were rejected, 13,338; enlisted, 2,726. Only 17 per cent. of the men offering, were received.

3,162	were	rejected	as	minors;
314	"	"	"	ruptured;
1,071	"	"	"	varicose veins;
732	"	"	"	over age;
630	"	"	"	unsound constitution;
1,965	"	"	"	intemperance.

If volunteers were subjected to as searching inspection, fewer would take the field, but they would be much more effective, because they would be less embarrassed by their hospitals, and would suffer less moral depression from seeing so many of their comrades stricken down by disease—the reason for which, they can not comprehend, so that every man fears he may be the next victim.

A most important sanitary precaution then for the surgeon to take, is to see to the integrity of body and mind of his men, before he passes them. For his own instruction on this point, he should carefully study the work of Henderson, or that published by the authority of the war department, for the guidance of recruiting officers of the army, by one of the authors of this work.

Pure air, one would suppose, could always be commanded in camp—but the fact is far otherwise, without great vigilance.

There is no circulation of air, or at least a very insufficient one, in the company tents. The men would never strike them, if they were not ordered. Six or eight men sleeping in a common tent, will render the air poisonous by morning. During the day it will be very imperfectly ventilated. What is to create any current of air through it? Is it surprising that men, passing night after night, in such an atmosphere, should get sick?

Again, men, particularly raw troops, will carry provisions from the messes into their tents, the remains of which are left to decompose upon the tent floor, or hang upon the tent poles. If the men are furnished with straw, they will never turn it out of their tents to expose it to sun, or purify it in any way, if *left to themselves.* All these things should be looked after by the medical officer, and he should make written suggestions, to the commanding officer, for the correction of these sanitary errors, whenever he perceives them to exist. The straw should be turned out daily, in dry weather, the tent thoroughly policed, and the tents struck at least once in three days.

It is of vast importance that the men's blankets and clothing should be frequently aired and repacked. Great care should be taken, that the men should sleep dry. Never let them lie down in wet clothes, if it can be avoided. The men always carry a change in their knapsacks. If they get soaked on a march, let them put on at least a dry shirt and drawers, after their tents are pitched, and dry their wet clothes by their camp fires.

A ditch should always be dug around a tent, sufficient to carry off any rain that may fall, so that the tent floor may be dry.

In selecting ground for a camp, unless uncontrollable strategic reasons compel, low moist ground is always to be avoided, no matter how attractive it may look. A dry gravelly soil is always to be preferred. Before determining upon the ground, a spade should be sunk a foot or more, to ascertain whether it is sufficiently drained to make it safe for the men to sleep on. For obvious reasons, the vicinity of marshes, particularly the leeward side of them, should be avoided, if possible.

When the camp is to remain more than a week, in the same place, bunks may be readily made for the sick, by driving forked stakes into the ground at the corners, laying side pieces in the forked ends, and then making transoms of the staves of flour barrels. It is advisable to do this whenever practicable. If men are well encamped and the camp well policed, the sick list will be very much diminished. Vaidy remarks, upon this point, that during a campaign one can not calculate upon less than 10 per cent. of sick, and fearfully more if badly encamped, badly provisioned, defeated, etc.

The subsistence of the men is a matter of the greatest importance, as regards quality, quantity, and mode of preparation. The importance of a full stomach to a soldier, has always been recognized. Frederick the Great, remarked, "a soldier's courage is in his stomach." A prudent general will always feed his soldiers before fighting, if he has the means. Men insufficiently fed fail, as soldiers, and more readily succumb to morbific influences. Both body and mind show the effects of a poor diet. The U. S. Army ration, however, is all sufficient for the men, and, if well cooked, will keep them healthy and vigorous. The medical officer should inform himself upon the principles of cooking the articles composing the ration, so that he may be able to instruct the regimental cooks upon this important point.

Dr. Taylor, the principal medical officer of the British Army, in the Crimea, has remarked, that since he has turned his attention to it, he thinks a competent surgeon should know how to cook, and that he should learn it in the first part of his medical education.

Beef and pork are the animal parts of the regular ration. In the war with Mexico, we sometimes used mutton instead of beef, as it was more readily procured. Beef, however, is the most nutritious animal food ordinarily accessible to the soldier. Its composition is identical with blood. But that it may be readily assimilated, it is important that it be well cooked. Soldiers on a march, or in camp, have the greatest propensity to fry their beef. This is the worst possible way in which it can be cooked. It causes a horny hardening of the surfaces of the pieces, preventing the due transmission and diffusion of heat through it, renders the fiber tough, so that it is never sufficiently masticated. Again, the action of heat upon the fixed oils or fat, always used in frying, is to render these substances particularly offensive to the stomach. Fats give off, when boiling, in addition to carbonic acid, and imflammable vapor, a part of the fatty acids, and a most acrid volatile principle (acroleine). The meat is thus deprived of important nutritive principles, and evolves others positively injurious to the stomach. In that admirable and complete system of Military Institutes prepared by General Scott, forty years ago, under the title of General Regulations for the Army, frying was prohibited in the army kitchens. The best mode of cooking the beef is to make it into soup. "It is soup," says Frederick, "that makes the soldier." But it takes longer to make soup than to fry—3½ hours being required for the former, and only 15 to 20 minutes for the latter.

The British government sent Soyer, the famous cook, to the Crimea, to see if he could not devise some means of improving the soldiers' messes. Soyer found the most preposterous processes of cooking in the soldiers' kitchen; he set about remedying them with great zeal, and was happily successful. He has published his Army Receipts, some of which I have tried in the kitchens at Newport Barracks, and have found them palatable, nutritious and economical. and I strongly recommend their use. I here insert some of the most useful:—

SOUP FOR FIFTY MEN.

Put into the boiler, 7½ gallons of water; fifty pounds of beef or mutton; three pounds of rice; eight pounds of fresh-vegetables; ten tablespoonfuls of salt; one tablespoonful of pepper. Simmer three hours, and serve, Skim off the fat, which, when cold, is an excellent substitute for butter.

PLAIN IRISH STEW FOR FIFTY MEN.

Cut 50 pounds of mutton into pieces of a quarter of a pound each; put them in the pan; add eight pounds of onions, twelve pounds of whole potatoes, eight tablespoonfuls of salt, three tablespoonfuls of pepper; cover all with water, giving about half a pint to each pound; then light the fire. An hour and a half of gentle boiling will make a most excellent stew. Mash some of the potatoes to thicken the gravy, and serve. Fresh beef, veal, or pork, will also make a good stew. Beef takes two hours doing.

This I know to be a most excellent dish. It can always be prepared upon the march, in time for the men's dinner or supper.

FRENCH BEEF SOUP—CAMP FASHION.

Put in the camp kettle, 6 lbs. of beef, cut in two or three pieces, bones included; ¾ lbs. of plain, mixed vegetables, as onions, carrots, turnips, celery, as can be obtained, or 3 oz. of desiccated vegetables; 3 teaspoonfuls of salt, 1 of pepper, 1 of sugar; 8 pints of water. Let it boil gently for three hours; remove some of the fat, and serve.

The addition of ½ lb. of bread, cut in slices, or 1 lb. of broken biscuits, well soaked in the broth, will make a very nutritious soup. This is enough for six or eight people. The quantity required for a company is easily calculated.

STEWED SALT BEEF AND PORK FOR ONE HUNDRED MEN.

Put in a boiler, of well soaked beef, 30 lbs., cut in pieces of ¼ lb. each; 20 lbs. pork, cut up; 1½ lbs. sugar; 8 lbs. onions, sliced; 25 quarts of water; 4 lbs. rice. Simmer gently for three hours; skim the fat off the top, and serve.

To soak the meat, it should be placed in camp kettles, well covered with water, and left to soak all night. If the water can be changed once or twice, it will be better. Prior to using, it should be washed and squeezed with the hands.

If soup is not made, the beef may still be boiled, but in a different way. Soup should be made by beginning the process with cold water. *Bouilli* by putting the beef into boiling water at first, and then simmering at 160° till done.

The general rule is, that roasting is to be done quickly, and boiling slowly.

In roasting, the loss of beef is, 19, mutton, 24, but their chemical constitution is not changed. The loss is made up of water evaporated, and fat melted and mixed with the gravy. But in boiling, the loss, though less in amount, is more serious in quality; it is made up of fat, gelatine and water, with some albumen and hematosine; and if salt is used, potash is likewise lost. Therefore the broth should be eaten.

The bean soup, made by soldiers in the army, is the best I have ever eaten. They prepare it by soaking the beans all night. The ration of pork is boiled in it. and any fresh or desiccated vegetables they can procure. Potatoes and onions are great favorites with them. It is seasoned to the taste with salt and pepper.

DRINKS.

Among European soldiers, water, beer, cider, wine and brandy are used. Ours use coffee and tea. Whisky was formerly issued daily to the troops; but this was abolished in 1832, and coffee and tea substituted. Recently a ration of whisky has been again authorized, upon a march, upon fatigue duty, and upon the frontiers.

Vaidy objects to hot drinks, such as tea and coffee, from their expensiveness and difficulty of preparation. He thinks they beget luxurious habits that must be interrupted on a campaign, He attributes the advice of the British surgeons to use them in malarious districts as prophylactics, rather to their national taste, than to the judgment of enlightened physicians.

Sir George Ballingall, on the other hand, says he saw the most marked effects from them in checking the extension of a malignant fever prevailing in the garrison at Hull. Dr. William Ferguson considers coffee or tea, in the morning, more indispensable than dinner, and regards them as sovereign against all the dangers of the morning—the cold, dampness, malaria, etc. I have no doubt of their great value, particularly in malarious districts. In tropical countries, a cup of hot coffee is the first thing, in the morning, with all who can afford it. I consider it imprudent for the surgeon to visit his hospital in the morning until he has taken his coffee.

If tea can be procured, I consider it preferable to coffee, in camp or on a march, because it can be much more easily prepared. Soldiers rarely succeed in making coffee clear and palatable under these circumstances. I insert Soyer's method of preparing both, as the best I know of.

COFFEE A LA ZOUAVE FOR TEN MEN.

Put 9 pints of water into a canteen saucepan, on the fire; when boiling, add 7½ oz. of coffee; mix them well together with a spoon or piece of wood; leave on the fire a few minutes longer, or until just beginning to boil. Take it off, and pour in 1 pint of cold water; let the whole remain 10 minutes, or a little longer; the dregs will fall to the bottom, and your coffee will be clear. Pour it from one vessel into another, leaving the dregs at the bottom; add two teaspoonfuls of sugar to the pint. If milk is to be had, make 2 pints less of coffee, and add that much milk; boiled milk is preferable.

TEA FOR EIGHTY MEN.

Put 40 quarts of water in a boiler to boil; place the rations of tea in a fine net, very loose, or in a large perforated ball; give one minute to boil; take out the fire, if too much; shut down the cover; in ten minutes it is ready for use.

WATER.

The water the men drink is of great consequence, and should be selected with as much care as possible. The quality of the water at hand should have great influence in the selection of camping grounds. Running streams are, ceteris paribus, always preferable to pools or tanks. Hard water is prejudicial to health. Its usual salt is sulphate of lime. Its usual effect is to cause constipation and disordered digestion, besides producing unfavorable effects upon the urinary organs. Vaidy says, an expensive barrack was built in Spain, near a supply of Gypsum water. The consequence was, the men were all taken sick with colic and indigestion, and the barracks had to be abandoned.

Sometimes, however, this kind of water seems to cause diarrhea; but then there are probably other purgative salts in combination with it. Such water, if we must use it, should always be previously boiled. The most ready tests of the quality of water upon a march are its agreeable taste and its power of dissolving soap readily. Soldiers upon a march commit great excesses in the *quantity* of water they drink. The men fill their canteens before moving in the morning; which is all right, as the water at the camp is generally good; but before they have made one fourth of the day's march it is all consumed, or has become unpalatable from exposure to the sun. At every stream they meet with, or pool of water, they will, if unrestrained, break their ranks rush to the water, fill their stomachs and refill their canteens. This process I have seen repeated in armies a dozen times in one day. I am persuaded this is a fruitful source of that scourge of all armies, camp dysentery. The practice is wisely forbidden by the regulations of the army; but it is a very difficult habit to break up. Every exertion should be made by the medical officers to impress upon officers and men the necessity of self-denial in this respect, if they wish to preserve their health. I would recommend, whenever it is practicable, to fill the canteens with tea instead of water, or to add a ration of whisky to the water in the canteens.

In cold or wet weather, on guard, on fatigue duty, on the march, or whenever unusual exertion is to be made, I am persuaded the use of brandy or whisky is beneficial. They are food for the lungs, they retard the metamorphosis of tissue, and thus preserve, or rather, husband strength. Their protracted use, however, will be found prejudicial to health, as they obstruct the normal changes. Brandy is the most exceptionable in this respect. Whisky is much less so.

Whenever a camp is pitched in a peopled part of a country, it is immediately besieged by a host of pie and fruit dealers, whisky or beer sellers, and the like. The surgeon should earnestly urge upon the commanding officer the necessity of prohibiting this trade. It will certainly fill his hospital, if permitted to be carried on. No food or drink should be suffered to be introduced into the camp without having been previously inspected and approved by the medical officers. Soldiers require variety in their diet as much as other people, and this should be encouraged as far as practicable. Fresh vegetables, when they can be had, are always desirable additions to the messes. *Ripe* and fresh fruit may generally be used in *moderation*, without serious prejudice to health; but I am quite sure it would be better to do without them altogether in camp than to risk the consequences of the men indulging in unripe and stale fruit, if they are allowed fruit at all.

For the sick in hospital, of course a very different diet will be required. It is of great importance that this diet should be palatable, nutritious, and suitable to the impaired digestive powers of the sick. I have selected several of Soyer's receipts for the preparation of food for hospitals, which I subjoin. Some of them can be prepared in almost any situation or climate. A little ingenuity can adapt them to any situation in which war troops will be likely to be placed.

SEMI-STEWED MUTTON AND BARLEY.

Put in a convenient-sized caldron, 130 pints of cold water; 70 lbs. of meat, or about that quantity; 12 lbs. of plain mixed vegetables (the best that can be obtained); 9 lbs. 6 oz. of barley; 1 lb. 7 oz. of salt; 4 oz. of flour; 1 lb. 4 oz. of sugar; 1 oz. of pepper. Put all the ingredients into the pan at once. except the flour; set it on the fire, and when beginning to boil, diminish the heat, and simmer gently for two hours and a half; take the joints of meat out, and keep them warm in the orderly's pan; add to the soup your flour, which you have mixed with enough water to form a light batter; stir well together with a large spoon; boil another half hour, skim off the fat, and serve the soup and meat separate. The meat may be put back into the soup for a few minutes to warm again prior to serving. The soup should be stirred now and then while making, to prevent burning or sticking to the bottom of the caldron.

The joints are cooked whole, and afterward cut up in different messes; being cooked this way, in rather thick stock, the meat becomes more nutritious.

Note. The word "about," is fixed to the half and full diet, which varies the weight of the meat; but ½ lb. of mutton will always make a pint of good soup; 3 lbs. of mixed preserved vegetables must be used, when fresh are not to be obtained, and put in one hour and a half previous to serving, instead of at first. They will then show better in the soup, and still be well done.

All the following receipts may be increased to large quantities, but by all means follow the weight and measure:

BEEF SOUP.

Proceed the same as for mutton, only leave the meat in till serving, as it will take longer than mutton. The pieces are not to be above 4 lbs. weight, and for a change, half rice may be introduced. The addition of 2 lbs. more will make it thicker and more nutritive. ¼ lb. of curry powder will make an excellent change also. To vary the same, half a pint of burnt sugar water may be added; it will give the soup a very rich brown color.

BEEF TEA.

Cut 3 lbs. of beef into pieces, the size of walnuts, and chop up the bones, if any; put it into a convenient-sized kettle, with ½ lb. of mixed vegetables, such as onions, leeks, celery, turnips, carrots (or one or two of these, if all are not to be obtained); 1 ounce of salt; a little pepper; 1 teaspoonful of sugar; 2 oz. of butter; ½ pint of water. Set it on a sharp fire for ten minutes or a quarter of an hour, stirring now and then with a spoon till it forms a rather thick gravy at bottom, but not brown; then add 7 pints of hot or cold water, but hot is preferable; when boiling, let it simmer gently for an hour; skim off all the fat, strain it through a seive, and serve.

THICK BEEF TEA.

Dissolve a good teaspoonful of arrowroot in a gill of water, and pour it into the beef tea twenty minutes before passing through the seive.

MUTTON AND VEAL TEA.

Mutton and veal will make a good tea by proceeding precisely the same as above. The addition of a little aromatic herbs is always desirable. If no fresh vegetables are at hand, use 2 oz. of mixed preserved vegetables to any of the above receipts.

CHICKEN BROTH.

Put in a stewpan, a fowl; 3 pints of water; two teaspoonfuls of rice; 1 teaspoonful of salt; a middle-sized onion, or 2 oz. of mixed vegetables; boil the whole gently for three quarters of an hour; if an old fowl, simmer from one hour and a half to two hours, adding one pint more water; skim off the fat, and serve. A small fowl will do.

Note. A light mutton broth may be made precisely the same by using a pound and a half of scrag of mutton instead of fowl.

For thick mutton broth, proceed as for thick beef tea, omitting the rice; a tablespoonful of burnt sugar water will give a rich color to the broth.

PLAIN BOILED RICE.

Put two quarts of water into a stewpan, with a teaspoonful of salt; when boiling add to it ½ lb. of rice, well washed; boil for ten minutes, or till each grain becomes rather soft; drain it into a colander, slightly grease the pot with butter, and put the rice back into it; let it swell for about twenty minutes near the fire, or in a slow oven; each grain will then swell up, and be well separated; it is then ready for use.

SWEET RICE.

Add to the plain boiled rice, 1 oz. of butter, 2 tablespoonfuls of sugar, a little cinnamon, a quarter of a pint of milk; stir it with a fork, and serve; a little currant jelly or jam may be added to the rice.

RICE WITH GRAVY.

Add to the rice 4 tablespoonfuls of the essence of beef, a little butter, if fresh, half a teaspoonful of salt: stir together with a fork, and serve.

ARROWROOT MILK.

Put into a pan 4 oz. of arrowroot, 3 oz. of sugar, the peel of half a lemon, ¼ teaspoonful of salt, 2½ pints of milk; set it on the fire, stir round gently, boil for ten minutes, and serve. If no lemons are at hand, a little essence of any kind will do.

When short of milk, use half water; half an ounce of fresh butter is an improvement before serving. If required thicker, put less milk.

THICK ARROWROOT PANADA.

Put in a pan 5 oz. of arrowroot, 2½ oz. of white sugar, the peel of half a lemon, a quarter of a teaspoonful of salt, four pints of water; mix all well, set on the fire and boil for ten minutes; it is then ready.The juice of a lemon is an improvement; a gill of wine may also be introduced, and ½ oz. of calf's foot gelatine previously dissolved in water will be strengthening. Milk, however, is preferable if at hand.

RICE WATER.

Put 7 pints of water to boil; add to it 2 oz. of rice washed, 2 oz. of sugar, the peel of two thirds of a lemon; boil gently for three quarters of an hour, it will reduce to 5 pints; strain through a colander, it is then ready.

The rice may be left in the beverage, or made into a pudding, or, by the addition of a little sugar or jam, will be found very good for invalids.

BARLEY WATER.

Put in a saucepan 7 pints of water, 2 oz. of barley, which stir now and then, while boiling, add 2 oz. white sugar, the rind of half a lemon thinly peeled; let it boil gently for about two hours, without covering it, pass it through a sieve or colander—it is then ready. The barley and lemon may be left in it.

TOAST AND WATER.

Cut a piece of crusty bread about ¼ lb. in weight; place it upon a toasting-fork, and hold it about six inches from the fire, turn it often, and keep moving it gently until of a light yellow color; then place it nearer the fire, and when of a good brown chocolate color, put it in a jug and pour over 3 pints of boiling water, cover the jug until cold, then strain it into a clean jug and it is ready for use. Never leave the toast in it, for in summer it would cause fermentation in a short time. This will keep good some time in bottles.

Baked apple toast and water.—A piece of apple, slowly toasted till it gets quite black, and added to the above, makes a very nice and refreshing drink for invalids.

Apple rice-water.—Half a pound of rice, boiled in the above until in pulp, passed through a colander, and drink when cold.

All kinds of fruit may be done in the same way. Figs and French plums are excellent, also raisins. A little ginger, if approved of, may be used.

Apple barley-water.—A quarter of a pound of pearl barley, instead of toast, added to the above, and boil for one hour, is also a very nice drink.

Citronade.—Put a gallon of water on to boil; cut up one pound of apples, each one into quarters, two lemons in thin slices, put them in the water, and boil them until they can be pulped; pass the liquor through a colander; boil it up again with half a pound of brown sugar, skim, and bottle for use, taking care not to cork the bottle, and keep it in a cool place.

For Spring drink.—Rhubarb, in the same quantities, and done in the same way as apples, adding more sugar, is very cooling. Also green gooseberries.

For Summer drink.—One pound red currants bruised with some raspberry; half a pound of sugar, added to a gallon of cold water, well stirred, and allowed to settle.

Mulberry.—The same, adding a little lemon peel: a little cream of tartar or citric acid added to these renders them more cooling in summer and spring.

Plain lemonade.—Cut in very thin slices three lemons; put them in a basin; add half a pound of sugar, either white or brown; bruise all together, add a gallon of water, and stir well. It is then ready,

French plum water.—Boil three pints of water; add in six or eight dried plums previously split, two or three slices of lemon, a spoonful of honey or sugar; boil half an hour and serve.

For fig, date, and raisin-water, proceed as above, adding the juice of half a lemon to any of the above. If for fig-water, use six figs.

Any quantity of the above fruits may be used with advantage in rice, barley, or arrowroot-water.

The medical officer should *generally* upon the march, and *always* during an action, carry upon his person, a case of pocket instruments and a canteen of good brandy or whisky. Wounded mēn frequently require a mouthful or two of stimulus for the relief of the shock, that in a greater or less degree, follows the receipt of a gun-shot or other wound.

CHAPTER III.

CAMP—DYSENTERY.

I CONSIDER the various forms of Dysentery, or Diarrhea, that prevail in camp, as being so intimately related to each other, it would serve no good purpose to treat of them separately. Sir George Ballingall treats of them under the title of Tropical Dysentery. The different features the various forms present, are probably due to climate or other accidents. Their prevalence and fatality in armies has always been marked; I have never known troops in campaign to escape it. It undoubtedly differs from ordinary dysentery in many respects. Thus Pringle remarks: "it is least known out of the field, and often general and fatal there." There were 23,000 cases in the Peninsular army, and nearly 5,000 deaths. It is most prevalent and fatal in hot climates. In India, the deaths from this disease are double those from fevers. In the Florida war, in 1836, it was most extensively prevalent and fatal; and the same is true of the Mexican war; and there the deaths from it, among the new troops, were double those of the old army. Its causes are principally violations of the laws of hygiene I have treated of in the preceding Chapter. I am confident, from my own observations, it may be very materially controlled by a due attention to these. Sir George Ballingall assigns, as the remote causes, heat combined with moisture; immoderate and indiscriminate use of fruits; abuse of spiritous liquors; exposure to currents of wind, and night dews.

Pringle refers, also, to heat and moisture as remote causes, and observes, that seasons favorable to the generation of flies, caterpillars, and other insects, whose increase depends upon corruption, are most productive of dysentery. Rush coincides in this opinion, and says, the remark applies equally to bilious fevers, and has often been verified in Philadelphia. Pringle also remarks upon the similarity of the causes, remote and exciting, of malarial fever and dysentery, and says of the men exposed to the same causes, some get one, some the other, and some both — such as after fatigue upon a hot day, sleeping upon the damp ground, or in wet clothes.

This is one of the most prolific causes of camp dysentery, and one to which raw troops are particularly exposed. The regular soldier, upon his arrival at the ground selected for the camp, will relieve himself of his knapsack and arms, and then, while waiting for the train with the tents, etc., will collect wood for the camp fires. When the train comes up, he attends to the pitching of his tent, the preparation of his evening meal, washing his feet, drying his clothes, etc. When everything is done, he lies down and passes a comfortable night. The raw recruit, on the other hand, will throw himself on the ground as soon as he halts—perhaps go to sleep, get thoroughly chilled, puts off his preparations for the night until the last moment, and, in consequence, has a badly-cooked meal and an uncomfortable tent, imperfect sleep, and rises for the next day's march but slightly refreshed. I point out this error that it may be hereafter avoided.

Pringle considers camp dysentery to be contagious, though he admits the infection to be less virulent than small-pox or measles. He says: "In camp, the contagion passes from one who is ill, to his companions in the same tent, and from thence, perhaps, to the next. The foul straw becomes infectious. But the great source of infection seems to be the privies, after they have received the dysenteric excrements of those who first fall ill."

Copland mentions the "fruit of hot climates, from his own observation and that of others," as a frequent cause. In my opinion, the fruit of all climates, indiscriminately used, will very generally excite it. There was a notion prevailing at Tampico, while I was there, that the banana was a remedy for it, though the inhabitants say that a drink of brandy, after eating bananas, is sure to make one sick. My observation does not confirm the innocuousness of the banana I had, myself, a severe attack of dysentery from a moderate indulgence in this fruit. I have seen, also, a number of cases excited by the use of the fresh limes so abundant at Acapulco, on the Pacific. Copland enumerates, among the causes, "badly-cooked meat or other food; pork; sour or bad wine; minute insects or their ova or animalcules in the water used for drink." "Several agents determine inflammatory irritation of, and an inordinate flux of fluids to the mucous surface of the large intestine, and their usual results" . . . . "exposure to cold, or cold and moisture, especially during or after great atmospheric warmth."

"Suppression of the secretions and excretions, poured into the large bowels, especially the biliary fluid, and accumulation of mucus in the follicles, are not altogether without effect in causing or prolonging the disease, especially of some of its protracted states; and several of the exciting agents, particularly cold, moisture, and malaria partly act in this way."—(Copland). Copland then gives the causes that disorder, or, as it were, corrupt these secretions and the circulating fluids—"unripe fruit, blighted grain, flesh and viscera of diseased animals, water holding putrid animal and alkaline substances in solution. They exert a septic action upon the mucous surface, the circulation, and, ultimately, the soft solids."

He also notices the convertibility of malignant fevers and dysenteries, by the concurrence of the exciting causes of the latter with the causes of the former. The causes that have most impressed me as exciting the disease are, in addition to the influence of cold and moisture, suppression of secretion, the cutaneous especially; errors in diet; neglect of ventilation of tents, quarters, and straw; drinking impure, or too much, water; bad police of camp; infection from the men's sinks. I must say a word or two upon the last.

In regular encampments, the place for the men's sinks is one hundred and fifty paces in front of the color line—those of the officers, one hundred paces in rear of the train. But when convenient, the regulations allow the sinks of the men to be placed in rear or on a flank. Both are to be concealed by bushes. Now, in my opinion, the choice of these places should be determined by the direction of the prevailing winds at the place of encampment, so that the offensive effluvia shall be carried away from the camp. There is no doubt, in my mind, that dysentery has been frequently increased, in camp, by a neglect of this precaution. The usual method of constructing these sinks, is to dig a shallow trench, some eight or ten feet long, to drive a strong forked stake at each end, and to place a strong pole, from one fork to the other, for the men to sit on. These sinks should be at least five feet in depth; immediately after reveille, not less than six inches of earth should be thrown upon the deposits of the preceding day and night, and when they are filled to within two and a half feet of the surface, they should be completely filled up and new sinks dug. If it can be procured, I would strongly recommend the following disinfectant, as cheap and effective, for use both in camp and hospital sinks; I have transcribed it from the last volume of the Annual of Scientific Discovery:

Sulphate of iron and alum are dissolved in water, till the solution is of the strength of 55°, it is then evaporated for 8 or 10 hours, during which 8 or 10 per cent. of lime is mixed with the compound—

it is evaporated to a hard compact cake, finally run into forms, and exposed to the air till it is perfectly dry, then reduced to powder. It may be kept in this form, or in solution; it has no odor. It instantaneously disinfects putrifying matter, privy vaults, etc.

There are many other circumstances, in addition to those I have already mentioned, that go to show a relationship between camp dysentery and malarial fevers. Johnson, in his work on tropical climates, says, in this disease the functions of the liver and skin, are always implicated. "He will defy any one who has carefully watched the disease, at the bedside, to produce a single instance in which these functions were carried on in a natural manner, at any period of the disease."

Sir Simon Howard, of the East India service, in an alarming epidemic of this kind, caused the men to be kept in barracks out of the sun, from 8 A. M. to 4 P. M., with the effect of diminishing the disease in a fortnight, and converting aggravated dysentery into common diarrhea. This shows the affinity between the acute dysentery or colonites, and the hepatic flux of Ballingall. It is the hepatic flux, however, that within my observation, has been most prevalent in our camps, and most prolific of the chronic cases.

Symptomatology.—There will be no difficulty of diagnosis in these cases. The symptoms of ordinary dysentery are well known—the most prominent of which, are more or less fever, frequent calls to stool, with griping and tenesmus, bloody and mucous dejections, small in quantity. But in camp dysentery, we have every degree of extreme disturbance, from the more violent forms of acute dysentery, to a trifling looseness or diarrhea. The alarm of the patient will be in proportion to the violence of the attack; still there is no grade not liable to run into fatal disorganization of the bowel. The security frequently felt from the trifiing nature of the attack, may betray the patient into fatal neglect. A prudent surgeon will watch closely the habits of the men, and interfere at once when he finds a soldier running too frequently to the sink. He will do well to walk along the line at the stated roll calls, and observe the sanitary expression of the men.

Sir G. Ballingall says, "the hepatic flux more frequently attacks those who, from habit or constitution, are less liable to violent inflammatory attacks, and more prone to irregular and disordered secretions of bile." These men are those of the nervous and melancholic temperaments; but I have found it as frequent in the sanguine, phlegmatic, and mixed temperaments, as any others. In fact, as far as my observation goes, we may take this form as the type, and refer all others to it; superadded causes determine the grade, either in excess or deficiency. It comes on very often as common diarrhea; the man complains that he has to go to the rear half a dozen times a day—he does not notice the character of the discharges—they vary in quantity, profuse or the reverse; next he will have griping and colicky pains about the umbilicus; then the discharges are unnatural, frothy, like yeast, too light in color; he is flatulent, loses his appetite, complains of "inward thirst," sometimes of nausea—his skin becomes dry, pulse quick. In the more chronic cases, the appetite is increased, and can not be restrained; the man emaciates rapidly, the tongue is furred, or of all colors, from white to the darkest bilious hue. Now, if the disease goes on unchecked, the appetite may improve, the tongue become cleaner, the fever less, but the flux continues, and emaciation goes on; the dejections assume, in their course, all sorts of appearances—serous, murcous, gelatinous, sometimes that of a uniform fluid feculent matter, more or less offensive, sometimes containing particles of food undigested. The older authors called those whitish particles, corpora penguia (Aretæus), σαρκεσ (Hippocrates). Pringle examined them in some of his cases, and found them to be particles of cheese. Copland notices that the discharges vary from a white albuminous, or white of egg appearance, to a dark olive green or greenish black; sometimes marbled, or on one day like chalk and water, and another like a dark jelly or green fat of turtle. Blood is often either so intimately mixed with the dejections, as to give them a uniform brick red color, or quite distinct and fluid, or partially coagulated. The discharges are sometimes as black and as thick as tar. The uniform brick, or darker red discharge, occurs frequently toward the close of life, and is apt to mislead the surgeon—it looks like an improvement in the character of the discharges, but it is generally a fatal symptom. Sometimes we have streaks of pus in the discharge.

We have increase of fever at night—the pulse becomes irregular, intermitting, frequent, weak; the tongue glazed, red, fissured, or like typhus; the skin harsh, dry—looks as if the man had not washed or changed his shirt for a month—the surface is scurfy or pulverulent; the emaciation is extreme, the ears transparent; eyes glassy; the lips white; the teeth covered with sordes; the lips retracted so as to show the teeth—cadaveric smell: syncope if the man is raised up; then, perhaps, low delirium for a day or two, and the man dies. Sometimes there is a cessation of the discharges for

24 or 48 hours—the man thinks he is beginning to mend—then an inclination to stool is felt, the man gets up, staggers to the vessel, falls over and is dead.

The urinary secretion is variously affected during the progress of the disease. In the earlier stages, it is not uncommon to have vesical irritation, with frequent micturition and diminished excretion. This is more common in the "colonites" variety; but in the latter stages the quantity of urine is normal, 30 to 40 ounces daily, but of a low specific gravity 1.002; this gives but 4.66 of solids in 1000, which is less than one tenth of the normal proportion. This may account for the typhoid symptoms we then see.

Pain is not constant in the progress of the disease; still pressure over the sigmoid flexure of the colon, will generally discover some tenderness, particularly in the earlier stages. In the progress of the case, the abdomen becomes hard and inelastic.

The duration of the disease is from a few days to four months. I have known acute dysentery prove fatal in 24 hours; death may come at any time, it will be governed by the severity of the attack, the character and seat of the original lesion; the powers of resistance in the constitution, etc. But camp dysentery is essentially chronic in its tendencies, I have known it to last for years, and the patient eventually recover; this, however, is rare.

Autopsies, in these cases usually reveal the omentum retracted to the arch of the colon, demented of fat, a mere shred; sometimes it is adherent to different portions of the intestine, but this is an accident due to local complication. The external coats of the intestine are scarcely altered—some slight change of color perhaps. Peritonitis from exhaustion may leave some traces here, but it is not common. The small intestine is distended with flatus; the large, contracted, sometimes as if strictured. Parts of it give a sense of thickness, as if swollen, particularly about the sigmoid flexure, and occasionally the appendix vermiformes. The colon is frequently adherent to the other viscera. Sometimes, in the rapid cases, the disintegration of the inner coats extends through the peritoneal coat, so that the gut is torn asunder in running it over in the usual way. But when the intestine is laid open, extensive destruction is disclosed; ulcers of all sorts and sizes stud the large intestine, clustered more especially about the sigmoid flexure, but extending throughout it, and frequently passing into the ilium. Inflammation of the mucous coat of all the small intestines is not unusual. Sometimes the ulcers are raised, and their bases indurated. Again extensive sloughing of the mucous and submucous coats is seen, and the intestine gets torn by the slighest strain, even by its own weight. Invagination is occasionally met with, or perforation of the intestine, inducing fatal peritonitis.

The remaining viscera rarely escape; the most frequent complications are those of the liver, next of the spleen; the pancreas is occasionally involved. That the gall bladder should contain viscid black bile is to be expected, and also that the mesenteric glands should partake of the irritation of the corresponding portions of the intestine.

Johnson thinks the liver complication an essential part of the disease. O'Brien investigated this point carefully in an extensive epidemic in Ireland, and found the liver involved in one half of the cases only, the spleen in one quarter, the small intestine in two thirds, the colon and rectum in all. Abscess of the liver is not so common as Johnson supposed. In India it may be due to other causes, such as engorgement of the gland from climate and diet. In Mexico, it is very common among intemperate pulque drinkers.

The symptoms and morbid appearances show the disease to be one of the chylopoetic viscera, *sometimes* involving them all, and *always* the intestinal canal, *i. e.* leaving there indications of the most destructive structural changes. That the disease is essentially inflammatory, seems to have been the prevalent notion of its nature. Pringle is inclined to that opinion, and Ballingall expresses it emphatically. I think it decidedly congestive. Copland is the first author I know of to admit this, but with caution, and many qualifications. He, however, says finally, in speaking of hepatic flux: "In most such cases, and in many of the simple as well as the most severe forms, congestion of the portal vessels and obstructions of this part of the circulation, are concerned in the production and perpetuation of the dysenteric symptoms."

This, in my opinion, is always the point of departure of camp dysentery. Suppressed or vitiated secretion is its first result, and these act and react on each other, and we have fullness of the vessels, or over-distention, resulting in the destruction of their elasticity, in both liver and intestine. This must be relieved somehow, either by nature or art, or it goes on to inflammation, and this the more intense the further the diseased part from the heart. This view is fully justified by a consideration of the most important recognized causes: suppression of the cutaneous transpiration, throwing the fluids upon the center; malarial infection, whether from the animalculæ of Kircher and Linnæus or the cryptogamous spores of Mitchell; venous plethora, from too much water, or water containing putrid infusoria; abuse of fruits; use of provisions of bad quality, or badly cooked, etc. The error has been in considering the flux to be the grand feature in the disease, whereas this is only symptomatic of more important and remote disturbance.

In camp dysentery, the patient seems eventually to perish of the combined effects of inanition and exhausting flux, analogous, at least, to hemorrhage. So long as his fat suffices for respiration, he may survive, emaciation constantly progressing, but beyond this limit, he fails. I may here remark that whatever may be the temporary condition of the flux, and however hopeful the patient from its apparent diminution or suppression, so long as *emaciation* is progressing, the man is *not* getting better.

In my view, we have, then, in camp dysentery—

1st. Congestion of the portal system.

2d. Inflammation, particularly of the mucous coat of the large intestine, but sometimes involving other organs and tissues.

3d. Vitiated condition of fluids concerned in assimilation of the food, with a consequent want of adaptedness of the latter to the wants of the economy.

4th. Probably paralysis of the lacteals and exhalents, so that the one does not take up the chyle, and the others pour out the thinner portions of the blood in abnormal and exhausting quantities, as well as sometimes the blood corpuscles themselves—indicating, moreover, serious implication of the ganglionic system in the assemblage of morbid phenomena.

Treatment.—The peculiar views of authors, and the prominent symptoms of the disease, have naturally suggested the treatment they recommend. Thus, the "inflammation" and "flux" notions would indicate astringents and antiphlogistics. Pain would call for anodynes, etc. Pringle, indeed, thought bleeding "unnecessary, yet conducive to the cure." "Still," he says, "unless the fever is kept up by inflammation not peculiar to the disease, *repeated* bleeedings are unnecessary and hurtful, as in most distempers arising from a putrid cause." In weakly habits and few feverish symptoms, he wholly omits that evacuation.

He speaks well of emetics, and used, in his early practice, wine of glass of antimony, which he had observed to be the best medicine in these cases, for relieving both stomach and bowels; but the roughness of its operation, and the prejudice against it among other officers, induced him to substitute ipecac. Still, among the common men, he added to this, one or two grains of tartar emetic. He observed that, whenever he gave the weaker or the stronger vomit, they were *most successful* when they *operated* by *stool*. The ipecac. treatment has been revived, of late, by Mr. Docker, surgeon of the 7th Royal Fusileers in the Mauritius. He says that, after repeated failures with other remedies, and a mortality of ten to eighteen per cent., he never fails with ipecac. in large doses. He had but one death in fifty, and that from abscess in the liver, the dysentery being completely cured! "In all constitutions, robust as well as delicate, the result is the same. In the very worst cases, when the strength of the patient is almost exhausted, after the whole range of remedies has been tried in vain, the disease running its course swiftly and surely to a fatal issue, 90 grains of ipecac. have been given, and forthwith the character of the disease, or, I should rather say, of the *symptoms*, has been entirely changed; for the disease itself is literally cured—put a summary stop to—driven out. The evacuations, from being of the worst kind seen in dysentery, have not *gradually*, not by any *degrees* however rapid, changed for the better; they have ceased at *once*, *completely*."

Mr. Docker uses an emetic, and sometimes a purgative first; then he applies a sinapism to the epigastrium, and gives ʒj tr. opii; and while the patient is under the influence of both, he gives the ipecac. in a draught or bolus. I find, however, from his cases, that this acted by procuring *good copious evacuations*, and that turpentine, camphor mixture, etc., were required for chronic mucous discharges in the after treatment.

Pringle always gave purgatives; if the stools were not copious enough with his ipecac., he gave calomel and rhubarb. After purging, he gave an opiate at night; but he says, it is better to omit opiates altogether, than to give them before purging, "for, though they seem to give relief, yet, by confining the wind and corrupted humors, they tend to fix the cause, and render the distemper more obstinate in the end." Herein he differs, reluctantly, from Sydenham, who, though he did not omit purging in *epidemic* dysentery, yet, at all other times he trusted to laudanum alone. Now whatever," says Pringle, "was the nature of those fluxes which he treated in that way, I must believe that such as are most incident to an army are of a less tractable nature, and, in general, can not be cured without repeated evacuation."

Sir George Ballingall says that *bloodletting* is the remedy upon which we must rely in the worst form, and in the inflammatory stages of dysentery; but he confesses that this opinion is grounded more upon the post-mortem appearances than upon any repeated or extensive experience of its beneficial effects upon the living.

Bampfield, also, insists upon bloodletting, but says, a large proportion of the practitioners in both Indies, not only discountenance the practice, but have never employed it. So Twining says, the cure of acute cases, in plethoric subjects, should be attempted by the early and free use of the lancet. But he naively adds, after each general bleëding, twelve or fourteen leeches should be applied to the abdomen, when pressure reveals pain. Others recommend bleeding to be pushed ad deliquium; and the further we go back, the stronger is the testimony as to its necessity.

Of course, all these authors refer to the semi-acute form of dysentery, in so strongly urging the use of the lancet; none of them would have thought of employing it in an ordinary case of hepatic flux.

Johnson and Annesly give calomel to the extent of one scruple to gr. ij. or gr. iij. of opium in twenty-four hours. Ballingall disapproves of this practice, in acute cases, but gives strong testimony to its efficiency in chronic hepatic flux, and pushes it to ptyalism; whenever the exhaustion of the patient does not forbid, he perseveres with it until the natural secretions are procured. Profuse salivation he condemns, as increased relaxation and debility are induced, and the patient is rendered incapable of taking the little sustenance he might be inclined to.

The limit I have imposed upon myself will not permit me to follow Copland, through the elaborate therapeusis he has developed for the many varied forms of the disease and the symptoms it may from time to time present; they are all referable to, and deducible from, the same principles of local inflammation; vitiated secretion, and perverted ganglionic and animal nervous function being the pathological condition. My own observation and experience, extending now over a period of thirty years, have convinced me that, with proper attention to military hygiene, though we may not succeed in completely preventing the occurrence of camp dysentery among troops in the field, still, we can so limit its prevalence as to make it no longer formidable. In treating of the causes of the disease, I have endeavored to point out the hygienic errors men commit, and thus afford the means of obviating or avoiding them. To carry out effectively the sanitary precautions I have indicated, the medical officer must endeavor to avail himself of the assistance of the officers of the regiment, and especially of the company officers. He should point out to them the necessity of watching over the habits of their men, on the march and in camp; of warning them against the consequences of infractions of the sanitary law, and of interposing their authority to prevent them from indulging in any of the practices we have endeavored to show are so prolific in inducing the disease in question.

When a man is attacked with any of the forms of camp dysentery, my constant practice is to give at once a purgative dose of sulphate of magnesia ʒj. combined with ¼ to ½ a grain of tartar emetic. If this does not procure copious catharsis, I repeat the dose the next day or the day after. My object is to unload the portal vessels, as well as to remove any irritating matters that may be present in the intestinal canal.

This being done, absolute rest is enjoined, and abstinence from all fluids for the next 24 hours. A spoonful or two of water at a time, to moisten the mouth, are all that should be allowed. At night, if the patient is restless, a few grains of Dover's powder will generally procure him a comfortable sleep. I have treated hundreds of cases successfully with no other medication, and I firmly believe that, in the great majority of cases of hepatic flux, no other remedies will be required. They may require, some of them, two or three days' abstinence from fluids, with rest, and a repetition of the saline cathartic, but these cases will not become chronic. When the symptoms are more severe, the case more obstinate, with pain and tenderness of the abdomen, after the purgation, I use, according to severity of symptoms, dry or wet cups to the abdomen, particularly over the sigmoid flexure of the colon. This I repeat from day to day, to keep up a constant counter-irritation upon the surface, by the one, or to institute an effective local depletion with the other. In acute dysentery with bloody flux, the cups can not be too thoroughly applied. I have not mentioned leeches, because they can not be procured in camp. When there is much symptomatic fever, with dry skin, I have sometimes been obliged to use small doses of ipecac. or Dover's powder, to determine to the surface, but always after the preliminary evacuations. Opiates and astringents, in the beginning of the treatment, are worse than useless. They cause the loss of valuable time, lull one into a false security, aggravate the congestion already existing, and frequently convert a perfectly manageable disturbance of the economy into a formidable and intractable disease.

In the more purely dysenteric cases, when the rectum is the chief seat of local difficulty, anodyne injections have long been favorite remedies. I can not say that I have seen any decided benefit from them. They do seem to allay tenesmus for a while, and thus procure some little rest to the patient; but from their frequent repetition, they become themselves sources of irritation, aggravate the sufferings of the patients, and are, of necessity, abandoned. I can not speak much more favorably of injections of nitrate of silver. The relief that follows them is only temporary—they do not cure; still, when the sufferings of the patient are so atrocious as they sometimes are in the acute form of dysentery, any means of even a temporary respite should certainly be put in requisition. The diet, in these cases, should of course be very simple, bland and unirritating, but nutritious. A few spoonfuls of thick rice water, or of strong animal broth, free from fat, and without seasoning, or of essence of beef, may be given several times in the course of the day; but the less water the patient drinks, the better.

One thing I neglected to mention in its proper place; and that is, the practice of soldiers, after a hot day's march, or in a southern climate, where the nights are almost always cool, to strip up their shirts, leaving the legs and abdomen bare, when they lie down for the night; nothing is more refreshing to the senses, and nothing more prejudicial to the health. I believe it to be the exciting cause of a great many of these cases of camp dysentery.

In spite, however, of any system of treatment, some cases of camp dysentery will become chronic, and are then of most difficult management. Once fixed upon an unfortunate patient, the chances are fearfully against his recovery. A few have constitutions sufficiently vigorous to react and recover, after even years of suffering.

Within the last five years, I have been more successful, however, in the treatment of these cases, and will now endeavor to give, in as few words as possible, the means I have employed.

In the purely dysenteric cases, after the subsidence of the fever, the bloody and mucous discharges still continuing, Hope's mixture has seemed to meet the indications well, as a constitutional remedy. As a local means, enemata of persulphate of iron, ten grains, in half an ounce of thin arrowroot, repeated three or more times a day, have been followed by the best results. Sometimes a few drops of laudanum may be added—half a drachm or less.

Absolute rest in bed is very essential. Dry cups to the abdomen, I use constantly; wet cups occasionally, when there is any tenderness to be discovered over the sigmoid flexure of the colon.

Massola, of the Sardinian army in the Crimea, found the use of ergotine in chronic dysentery, a very successful remedy. He gave ½ a grain hourly till the discharges were arrested. I have used this remedy since, in several cases, and have been pleased with the results. Sometimes, however, it has failed. I would recommend that it should be tried. In the chronic forms of the hepatic flux, it will perhaps be more useful than in the bloody and mucous fluxes.

Some three years ago, my friend Dr. Foster, of Cincinnati, mentioned to me, that he had seen surprising results in a case of chronic diarrhea, from the use of very small doses of Fowler's solution. I lost no time in testing its powers. The first case in which I employed it was, one of an old friend, a general officer in the army, who was the subject of a debilitating and harrassing diarrhea, contracted in Florida many years since. He kept it somewhat in check by the constant use of astringent and anodyne draughts. I gave him five drops of the solution a day, in divided doses, with the result of procuring an undisturbed night's sleep, for the first time in several months, and his complete recovery in a few weeks. I have since employed it in several cases, and always with more benefit than any other remedy I have ever used.

The perchloride of iron has been extravagantly lauded in all mucous fluxes, in a recent work by Deleau. He makes a solution of the salt, which he terms his normal solution, and which is of the strength of 30° Reaumur. Of this he makes a mixture with simple syrup, of 1 part to 60, and the dose is a teaspoonful. I have used the officinal solution in doses of ten drops, in a teaspoonful of syrup or water, and with good effect. It is worthy of a trial.

I have brought these remedies forward, because I believe them to be new in army practice, because I have seen good results from them, and because I have no confidence, whatever, in the whole catalogue of the other astringents, mineral and vegetable, that have been heretofore relied upon in the treatmet of chronic diarrhea.

Rest, dry cupping, and a bland but nutritious diet, with as little water drinking as possible; flannel worn habitually next the skin, well ventilated quarters, and protection from currents of air, are important adjuvants in the treatment of all the forms of chronic camp dysentery.

CHAPTER IV.

OF THE GENERAL HISTORY—CHARACTER AND TREATMENT OF GUNSHOT WOUNDS.

The phenomena of gunshot wounds differ, in so many respects, from those of other injuries, that it was for a long time supposed that this difference was due to the poisoning the balls. A similar notion was entertained by some of our officers, at Palo Alto, from the discovery that some of the Mexican balls were made of bell metal. Another of the earlier notions was, that the velocity of their projection through the air caused such a heating of their masses, as to convert them into cauterie, burning the tissues as they penetrated. Gale, a distinguished surgeon in the time of Henry VIII, wrote a book to prove both these notions untrue. The features of gunshot wounds, are due to the regular operation of natural laws, and neither artificial poisoning, nor the composition of the balls, has anything to do with their effects. From their first invention (which Monroe says was for the ruin of man), to the present day, many improvements have been made in firearms, to increase their destructive effects; but, although, great accuracy and surprisingly long range of fire have been attained, so that it would be supposed a body of infantry must be annihilated in approaching a battery well served, actual results do not verify any such calculations. More men were slain in battle in the old Greek and Roman wars, than at the present day. At the famous battle of Solferino, where rifled cannon and all the modern European improvements were used, the proportion of casualties to the forces engaged, was not as great as in our own battle at Molino del Rey, in the valley of Mexico. It is possible that the time of firing is less now than it was of old, but in considering a number of the best contested battles on record, I find that when the losses reach 33 per cent., the battle is ended. It seldom reaches anything like this figure—never more.

Projectiles, or other bodies inflicting wounds in battle, are generally buckshot, musket, pistol, or rifle balls, canister, solid or hollow round shot, grape, fragments of shell or stone, splinters from gun-carriages, etc. The latter cause lacerations and contusions, as well as penetrating wounds.

Of late years, the smooth bored muskets and spherical balls have fallen into disuse. The improved rifled barrels, and the conical ball have superseded them almost entirely. In the Crimea, all the small arms in use, except the Sardinian pistol, carried conical balls.

The weight of the English musket or rifle ball, is 1 oz. and 2 scruples—the Russian 1 oz. and 5 drachms, ours are 17 to the pound. The Russian ball is conical with a flat base, three rings and two raised ribs to fit the grooves in the barrel. Our balls are conical, with a cupped base and one ring.

In theory, the form of the conical ball is perfect. The grooves in the rifle, give it a gyratory motion round its axis, while the flange of the ring at the base, presented to the resistance of the air through which it is passing should prevent it from deviating from its plane of projection in any direction. But this pre-supposes that the density of the ball shall be equal throughout its mass, and that the plane of the ring shall be accurately and perfectly true, and normal to the surface of the ball; conditions that can not be secured, in the necessary mode of manufacturing these balls in large quantities. Accordingly, experiment has shown, that they strike a target in all possible directions, a circumstance that may account for the destruction inflicted by some of them, and which, I think, Macleod has erroneously supposed to be the general effect of the conical ball.

The Russian grape, range from one and a half ounces to three pounds—ours, one to six pounds. Canister are of all sizes, shapes, and irregular surfaces. Round shot vary from one to two hundred and ninety-four pounds. The last are for columbiads and sea coast defenses.

It will be readily conceived how different will be the effects from this great variety of projectiles; how all should differ from wounds inflicted by the old implements of war; and how multiform the characters of the injuries presented to the military surgeon. In my opinion, however, there is no reason to believe that the character or nature of the wounds we are likely to meet with in the present unfortunate disturbances, will differ in any essential feature from those with which we have been familiar with in former wars, from the fact that improved artillery and small arms will be, to some extent, employed. Should it prove otherwise, I have no doubt the resources of surgery will be fully equal to the emergency.

It would naturally be supposed that, when a ball projected with so much velocity, impinges upon any portion of the body, from the disproportion of the resistance to the power, it would pass onward in a right line; but there is no end to the eccentricities of their courses. A round ball has entered above the elbow on one side, and lodged in the opposite axilla. Another penetrated the right hip, and lodged in the left popliteal space. Balls penetrate the cavity of the thorax, and run round between the pleura and lungs without wounding the latter; and again, they have been known to pass round the abdominal parietes within the peritoneum without wounding the viscera.

Gulliver has reported a case in which the ball was found lodged in the posterior surface of the sternum, after entering at a distant part of the thorax. Hennen saw a man in whom a ball ran round the neck from one corner of the os hyoides to the opposite; another ascending a scaling ladder, received a ball in the center of the arm, it ran along the limb over the posterior part of the thorax, among the abdominal muscles, through the glutee, and presented in front of the middle of the opposite thigh. In another case, a ball passed between the shirt and skin, from the wrist to the shoulder, furrowing the skin, but without penetrating or flying off.

The irregular shape of fragments of shell, and the size of cannon balls, might be supposed always to inflict wounds, that could not escape recognition. Yet Macleod has recorded a case that occurred at Scutari, where a piece of a shell weighing three pounds had buried itself in a man's hip, making so small an opening that it was overlooked for three months, when it was extracted. Larrey reports a case in which a five pound ball was buried in a man's thigh, giving him no inconvenience except from the weight of the limb. Bégin has reported a similar case, in which the ball weighed nine pounds, and Hennen one in which a twelve pound ball was similarly buried, and only discovered after death.

The deflection of musket and rifle balls and the eccentricities of their courses among the muscles, etc., has been variously explained by different authors. Vidal thinks it due to the guns not having been methodically loaded, and thus the ball receives its impulse in the direction of a diameter not parallel to the axis of the piece, and hence will have a great tendency to deviate. I think if the supposition as to direction of original impulse is true, the direction of the ball would be corrected by the right cylinder through which it must pass before it escapes from the barrel, and that, therefore, Vidal's explanation is unsatisfactory. It moreover gives us no practical hint.

My own explanation is this: In the first place, if the ball does not strike in a direction normal to the surface of the body or limb, its tangential tendency, or tendency to deviate, will be equal to its momentum into the sine of the angle it makes with the surface. In the second place, after penetrating, with its new direction, it meets with various tissues of unequal density, elacticity and tension, which constitute a series of inclined or deflecting planes, opposing its passage, and causing it to deviate from a right line in all conceivable directions. Its velocity is constantly diminished as it passes on, until it escapes and falls to the ground, or is arrested among the tissues themselves. In this mode of considering the subject, it is not surprising that a ball should run round the neck instead of passing through, or that it should strike the anterior end of a rib and pass out near the spine, without traversing the lung.

Vidal has happily called the deviations "primary." He has given the name "consecutive deviations" to those which take place sometimes in the position of a ball lodged in the body in consequence of muscular action, change of posture of the patient, or of suppuration detaching it from its original point of arrest.

Balls impinging upon flat bones, are very frequently deflected.

Macleod says that conical balls are seldom deflected; that round balls pass spirally around the bones without breaking them, but that conical balls take the shortest course. He says that one of these balls passed through two men at Alma, and lodged in a third. There have been some curious calculations as to how many men a ball will pass through. Antonio says a 32-pound ball will pass through 70 men; an 8-pound ball, 40; a 1-ounce ball, 4. These are mere speculations, and not at all reliable.

In field works the upper part of the body is most exposed to shot; the defenses protect the lower part; hence the greater proportion of killed to wounded in field works than in the open field. The error in firing in the field, is generally that the piece is too much elevated, so that a great proportion of the balls projected pass over the heads of the opposing force; others, from other causes, fall short. It has always been a matter of great surprise to me that of the vast number of balls fired, so few should take effect.

Hennen calculates that of all gunshot wounds received in battle, there will be 2 in the abdomen, 4 in the neck or breast, 7 in the head, 10 in the arms, 4 in the hips or legs, 1 in the knee, and 2 in the feet.

Scrive has calculated from his observation in the Crimean war, that, in a siege, the distribution of wounds will be one third in the hip, one twelfth in the chest, and one fifteenth in the abdomen; in the open field, one tenth in the head, one twentieth in the chest, and one fortieth in the abdomen. The statistics of the positions of the wounds of those killed upon the field would be very interesting.

The sensation experienced from a musket wound is like that from a smart blow from a cane; if a bone is broken, the pain will be greater; if a joint is opened, both shock and pain will be still greater; if the thigh is broken, or a great cavity opened, the shock is severe, and particularly so if the abdomen is penetrated.

But sometimes, even in severe wounds, the pain is so trifling that the man is unconscious he is hit until he finds the blood trickling down the limb. Hennen, Macleod, and others, say they have known a limb shattered or carried away without the consciousness of the sufferer. Macleod says he knew an officer to have both legs carried away; he thought he had stepped into a hole, and was not aware of what had occurred to him till he attempted to rise.

The character of the wound will depend upon the weight, shape. and velocity of the missile, and the nature of the part wounded, Lacerated wounds result from fragments of shell or stone or splinters. As lacerations merely, there is no peculiarity about them; when complicated with penetrations, they partake of the character of gunshot or of bayonet wounds.

Macleod says, "a ball passing at great speed over the surface of a limb, may occasion a wound similar to that made by a knife. But this action of a ball is rare." I have never seen anything of this sort; it is possible, however, that the sharp flange of a conical ball or a sharp point upon the surface of a ball, might have this effect.

The character and gravity of a buckshot wound, will depend a good deal upon the distance of the object. Wire cartridges carry them close for 20 yards—at 50 they are more divergent—at 150 they will pass singly through a yellow pine board an inch thick. Shot wounds fired close are more dangerous than ball; it is singular how they distribute themselves in all directions among the soft parts, and what extensive disorganization they produce. Vidal remarks, that balls may traverse the lungs, making serious wounds, but the injury from shot is extensive and fatal. Round shot carry away limbs, and large flaps of the soft parts; they crush the bones and produce extensive braying of the viscera and muscles, sometimes without breaking the skin; but in these cases, the constitutional shock is fearful. A sergeant at Cerro Gorda had one buttock carried away by a round shot. This extensive wound granulated kindly and the man recovered without an untoward symptom. I once saw a leg carried away by a rifle ball, but it was discharged at a distance of only a few feet. The extensive concealed injuries produced by round shot, are very remarkable. Delpech records a case in which the bones of the leg were completely smashed, and still, fracture was not even suspected till after death. The liver has been torn to pieces and the lungs lacerated, while the skin has remained unbroken. Macleod has reported a case in which a man was hit by a round shot on the outer side of the right arm and thorax. There was a blue mark upon the arm, but none on the thorax. Death occurred in twenty hours. The peritoneal cavity was filled with dark blood, the right lobe of the liver was torn into small pieces, some of which were loose and mixed with the blood. There was no peritonitis, and the remaining viscera were healthy. Dupuytren mentions the case of a man wounded at the barricades in Paris. There was no sign of injury upon him, and his comrades suspected him of shamming. He was carried to the hospital and died. The muscles of one leg were found completely brayed, and still the skin was unbroken. An officer at the storming of Chapultepec while on horseback, had the calf of his right leg similarly injured; sloughing of the whole calf ensued, and yet this gentleman assured me he was totally unconscious of having received any blow upon the part.

These singular cases have been attributed to the windage of a passing ball; to the condensation of the air, occasioned by the ball in its passage, and its sudden expansion, afterward causing a rupture of the vessels; to electricity, generated by the passage of the ball through the air. These notions were long since exploded. An English surgeon as long ago as 1672, speaks of it as a thing not generally believed; he affirms, that a cannon ball passing ever so near can do no harm or no one above deck would escape. Epaulettes have been carried away from an officer's shoulder, and the wearer left unharmed. Death may be so sudden, in the part struck, as to give no time for the development of any external mark of injury. Larrey found so much internal disorganization in these cases, as to leave no doubt of actual contact. He, as well as Guthrie, supposes that balls have only a rectilinear motion in the first place, and they then carry away any part they touch; but that from the resistance offered by the air, and gravitation, they after a while acquire a motion around their axis, and then, with diminished velocity, they roll over a surface instead of carrying it away, and crush everything beneath. Vidal and Dupuytren suppose that balls have the two motions of rotation and progression *ab initio* and they thus roll over a surface or round a limb, crushing all underneath, without wounding the skin.

Gunshot wounds combine the characteristics of all other wounds, contused, lacerated, punctured, and incised. "Wounds from musket balls, particularly of the face, sometimes bleed considerably at the moment of injury, and for some little time afterward; although no large vessel shall be injured, to render the bleeding inconvenient or dangerous.

"When a limb is carried away by a cannon shot, any destructive bleeding usually ceases with the faintings and failure of strength, subsequent on the shock, and a hemorrhage thus spontaneously suppressed does not generally return; it is the effort of nature to save life." *

Wounds from musket or rifle balls are usually round, discolored at the entrance, and depressed—they are less regularly round at their point of exit, and the hole is larger there; the hole in the soft parts is usually less in diameter than the ball, the contusion at the point of entrance takes, as Sir Charles Bell remarks, the form of several concentric circles. At the center, the integument is killed, and sloughs about the size of the ball; sometimes a plug of the integument is carried in before the ball. In the next ring, the vitality of the integument is seriously compromised, but not entirely destroyed. It will depend upon circumstances whether it will be recovered or lost, such as the degree of ecchymosis, the subsequent inflammation, etc.

The next ring is composed of irritated and compressed tissue, and always inflames. Then there is a ring of simple bruising and discoloration of unequal extent and diffusion.

Vidal remarks, that it is in the third circle, that first movements toward reaction occur, as the parts there preserve their vitality, and are sufficiently irritated to excite inflammation. They swell and suppurate, and if the inflammation is kept within due bounds, the second zone may be saved, and only the eschar thrown off; this is always eliminated either entire or mingled with the pus. The es-

* Guthrie.

char does not extend throughout the whole track of the wound—there will probably be none at the point of exit. This is the type.

Sometimes there will be extensive sloughing and suppuration, and that of unhealthy pus; owing to the more extensive stunning of the tissues; to the nature of the tissues implicated such as the aponeuroses or fibrous tissues generally; to the bad constitution of the man, or his depressed morale; to the presence of pieces of clothing in the wound; to impure air, or bad food; or perhaps to endemic influence.

Sometimes the swelling and suppuration are so slight, that the wound seems to heal by the first intention. Ballingall mentions the case of a negro in India, who had a wound through the biceps muscle of the arm, which healed without suppuration. Macleod saw a wound through the gastrocnemius unite by the first intention on the fifth day. In hot climates, these exceptional cases are most frequent. If the incised wounds the effect of gunshot, of which Macleod speaks ever occur, this union, by the first intention, would be very probable, but I have never seen it. Vidal says he saw a wound implicating the knee joint, unite with so little suppuration, that he would have been deceived had he not watched the case very closely.

Larrey, Sanson, and Hunter, mention similar cases.

The wound at the point of exit usually heals first.

Different views as to the characteristics of entrance and exit holes, have been advanced by different observers. Macleod says, that the wound at the point of entrance is more regular and less discolored, than at the point of exit, but he is not so sure that the lips of the former are inverted, and of the latter, everted. If the speed of the ball is great, and there is no bone broken, there will be little difference in size or color—but if the speed be diminished, or a bone broken, the hole at the point of exit will be much larger, especially so with conical balls. But in close firing, and the speed of the ball undiminished, the difference is very small, and sometimes the entrance wound is the largest. He saw this twice. The general rule, I believe to be as first enunciated. Devirgie gives an instance in which the wound, at the point of entrance, was the largest, though the ball was fired at a distance. It is possible that this may occur, because an irregular ball may enter by its largest element, and escape by its smallest or the reverse—or the ball may be altered in its shape while traversing the limb, or it may carry in pieces of clothing, or of equipments, and thus modify the characteristics of wounds.

The holes made in bones, differ from those in the soft parts—in the spongy extremities of the long bones, they are sometimes similar to those in the soft parts, but in the flat bones, the hole is usually larger than the ball.

Inflammation and swelling always follow the wound in a short time; the lips of the wound become everted, then suppuration occurs, and the casting off of the sloughs with fever, sometimes severe, generally of the inflammatory, sometimes of the nervous or typhoid type.

Collapse, or shock, is, I think, an attendant of every wound. Sometimes it is appalling, and *may* indicate the gravity of the wound, but not always. Much depends upon the nerve of the man. It is greater in wounds of the lower extremities, than the upper, or if the wound is received while the man is standing. Chevalier says, it is greater if the ball strikes a muscle in action. It is always alarming in wounds, implicating the great cavities, the abdomen in particular. In some, it is soon recovered from; in others, it continues hours, and ceases only with life. It is relieved, if at all, by stimulants. Guthrie thinks, if it is persistent, it indicates severe internal injury. This may, perhaps, be so, if the external lesion is not sufficient to account for it, as in cases where the leg or thigh are carried off.

Collapse is marked by pallor of the surface, white lips, cold sweats, tremors, small and scarcely perceptible pulse—it is not likely to be mistaken.

The effects of balls, we have said, depend somewhat upon their shape. Macleod says, "the great velocity, peculiar shape and motion of the conical ball, give to its wounds a character considerably different from those present in wounds caused by round musket balls. If fired, at short range, and if it strike a fleshy part, the conical ball produces, I think, less laceration of the soft parts, than the old ball; but if the range be great, and parts struck bony, with little covering of flesh, as in the hand or foot, then the tearing, especially at the point of exit, is greatly more marked."

Now the effects of balls as hitherto observed upon bones, are, if they strike obliquely upon flat bones, they glance off, but even then they may be attended by dangerous results, particularly in the head; if they pass through a flat bone, the hole will be larger than in the soft parts. They sometimes strike the long bones, contusing, without breaking them, but producing death of the periosteum and consequent exfoliation, or abscess in the cavity of the bone; they may split the bone longitudinally without fracturing it, or even transversely without the fracture being complete; they may bury themselves in the spongy heads of the long bones without splitting them; I have seen a cavity of that nature in the head of the tibia; they may be deposited in the medullary cavities of the long bones, causing much mischief. Macleod says the conical ball always splits the bone in the direction of its axis downwards. It splinters and comminutes the bone in all directions, but is never split itself. Stromeyer, however, has reported a case in which a conical ball was split upon the patella; splitting the bone downward is not all peculiar to conical balls.

The nerves and blood-vessels generally very fortunately escape injury, unless the ball is ragged, or splinters the bones, or a limb or a large part of it is carried off. But sometimes an artery is perforated, as occurred to a young man in one of our large cities, a few years ago. In this case, the femoral artery was perforated by the ball with a part of the cylinders of the vessel left on each side of the opening. In this case, the vein was also injured. Both vessels were tied, but gangrene ensued and the patient died. Musket balls sometimes pass between an artery and its accompanying vein, without apparently injuring either. Inflammation and plugging of the vessels, however, is apt to ensue, with gangrene and the loss of the limb or life. Guthrie has given us an interesting case of this kind.

The phenomena of gunshot wounds, thus far noticed, I term the "constants," or the necessary phenomena. Others I term "variables," or accidents; these are either immediate or remote. The immediate are hemorrhage, and balls or other foreign bodies lodged in the wound. The remote are secondary hemorrhage, pyemia, traumatic erysipelas, hospital gangrene, and tetanus.

Treatment of gunshot wounds.—Hemorrhage, as an immediate accident of these wounds, is of rare occurrence. When it does occnr, of course it is necessary to secure the vessel or control the circulation through it by a tourniquet or compression at once. Whether the vessel should be tied or amputation of the limb resorted to, is a question I shall consider hereafter. If the former is the proper course, the bleeding aperture is a guide to the artery, and a ligature may be readily placed upon it. But if an artery of secondary importance is the one injured, and it can be readily compressed against a flat bone, the ligature will be seldom required. A graduated compress, charged with persulphate of iron, firmly applied *within* the wound, will, in most cases, effectually arrest the bleeding forever. In a case of this sort, I would not remove the compress until it was detached or loosened by suppuration. If the compress is resorted to in the continuity of a *limb*, the whole extremity should be bandaged, be ginning at the toes or fingers, as the case may be, and the limb afterward kept elevated.

When foreign bodies present themselves in the wound, they are to be removed as soon as practicable; but it is seldom that this can be done upon the field during the action. If either ball, broken bone, pieces of clothing, or anything else be within reach, it should be removed at once; but all wounds in which the presence of any of these substances is suspected, should be subjected to a thorough exploration after the man is removed from the field to the principal depot for the wounded at the rear.

The first dressings upon the field will be limited generally to cleaning the part well, applying a pledget of lint to the wound, and securing it with adhesive straps or a few turns of a roller. Guthrie objects to rollers, as they are so apt to get dirty or displaced; my objection to them is the inconvenience of their application and subsequent removal for systematic treatment. But sometimes we are compelled to use them. They should be cut off when removed for the thorough examination of the wound.

The first indication in the regular treatment is the removal of foreign bodies, and first of the ball.

Great differences of opinion have prevailed among military surgeons as to the necessity for removing the ball. There can be no question that they have sometimes remained for years without causing any serious inconvenience. Cysts, called by Balldeni, secondary cysts, form about them and enclose them, so that they are prevented from shifting their position, and need produce no further harm. But sometimes they remain for a time, and then suddenly excite an eliminative inflammation, and occasionally, though rarely prove fatal in the process, as by hemorrhage from ulcerative perforation of an artery, or by sudden change of place, as in the brain.

Dupuytren has called attention to the remarkable rapidity with which they sometimes change place, from change of position of the man, from muscular contraction, or from gravitation; and that these changes may produce immediate pressing symptoms.

Great importance is attached to the extraction of balls by most military surgeons. Hunter, however, has taken a different view of the subject, the rather, I am disposed to think, because his rival, Bell, urged this among his reasons for the more objectionable practice of debridement. The practical question is, do wounded men do as well with the balls remaining as when they have been extracted? Hutin examined 4,000 cases in the Hotel des Invalides, in whom the balls had been left unextracted. There were only 12 of these who suffered no inconvenience; 200 of the remainder had their wounds constantly opening and closing until the balls were removed.

Bégin insists that the indication for the extraction of the ball is always present, and it should be judiciously attempted. If we succeed, we have done much for the patient; if we fail, from fear of causing more mischief, or from insuperable obstacles, we have at least satisfied the demands of science. Macleod is very decided upon this point. He says that those in the Crimea who were for leaving the ball in, were the civil surgeons; the military surgeons were always for extraction. He asserts that patients who get along with them, are only exceptions; they invariably protract the cure, and increase the irritability of the patient.

The inconveniences arising from the presence of the ball, are, protracted suppuration; the blocking up of matter in the wound, causing burrowing abscesses; exfoliation of bone; ulceration of bloodvessels; tetanus, etc. Macleod says, that of four or five cases in which he could not find the ball, two died of tetanus. Now this fact is very suggestive; if there be any relation between tetanus and the presence of a ball, there would be no further dispute as to the necessity of removing it; it is very important to diminish the causes of this almost uniformly fatal accident.

Vidal can not agree with Hunter, as to the innocuousness of balls, and the power of nature to expel them as well as other foreign bodies; still, he is equally reluctant to advise protracted searches for them, particularly among delicate organs.

I think the weight of authority is all on one side, and have no doubt of its correctness. When a man is faint from loss of blood, from shock, or from the nature of the part wounded, so that any movement of his body might be followed by disastrous consequences, no one in his senses would think of turning him over, or anything else, to find out what had become of the ball; but the "*general rule is, as soon as practicable, to ascertain the position of the ball, and remove it as well as other foreign bodies, if it can be done without producing more mischief.*" Many balls present themselves near the surface, are easily felt, and readily extracted; but sometimes it is very difficult to ascertain their position. Probes may be used carefully, or gum-elastic bougies, for exploring the wound. If the wound is large enough, the finger is a very good probe. But, in cases of greater difficulty, the patient may be placed in the position he was in when he received the wound, putting the same muscles in action; while the surgeon places himself, as nearly as possible, in the direction of the projectile. Then consider, as Guthrie says, the "anatomy of the whole circle of injury"—the effect of the fasciæ, tendons, muscles, or bones in deflecting the ball, so as to judge of its probable course. The patient's idea of its course may give us valuable hints. Sir Charles Bell suggests the expedient of pressing along the course of the principal nerves of a limb, to ascertain the course of a ball—pain will be occasioned, frequently, in arriving over its site. It was Macleod's practice, after getting all the information he could from his patient, to give him chloroform, and then proceed with his exploration: he says he would risk much to get the ball out.

Mistakes of Diagnosis.—Stromeyer refers to a case where the head of the fibula and metatarsal bone were cut upon for a ball. Many similar mistakes might be mentioned. Statements of patients, that the ball has dropped out, are not always reliable; more than one may have entered; opposite orifices may have been made by different balls. In a battle cross fire is not uncommon, and the same man may receive two or three wounds at the same time, There can be no certainty except in exploration; or when opposite orifices have distinct characteristics of entrance and exit, I think they may be relied on. If the ball can be felt under the skin, or seen, it may be extracted at once, on the field; otherwise, it should be done at leisure, in the rear. Balls are very frequently easily detected after suppuration and subsidence of swelling. When flattened upon or wedged between bones, extraction is sometimes difficult, as in a case where I extracted from cervical spine. At the first dressing, all foreign bodies should be removed and the parts be well cleansed. Lint should then be applied and secured with adhesive straps, or a few turns of a roller. Guthrie objects to rollers: they get dirty, and are easily displaced. I object to them on account of the inconvenience of application and removal for systematic treatment, but it is frequently necessary to employ dressings during the removal of patients to the rear, when they may be cut off, if necessary.

Hospital Dressing.—Vidal says, poisoning being the predominant etiological idea, cauterization was naturally the principal indication in the treatment of the ancients. Parè changed this barbarous practice, and exposed its absurdities. He still, however, adhered to ointments—honey of roses, tinct. of myrrh, etc. These, however, are forgotten, and the modern question is between water dressings, hot or cold, and poultices, and simple lint, with or without a covering of cerate. The wound, I have said, is of a composite nature, and of every degree of severity. Its extremes are a simple contusion, and a braying of all beneath the skin. In the latter case, there will be little use for dressings. Amputation of a limb, first or last, must ensue. I was taught that a gunshot wound could not be poulticed too soon. This was Hunter's opinion. Now the fashion is *ice* altogether. The aim is to reduce the composite wound to a simple one, that union by the first intention may be effected as soon as possible. For this reason we amputate when a limb has been shot away. We remove the irregular flaps of soft parts. We try to diminish the extent of the traumatic surface, which is the closest approximation we can make to a simple wound in these cases. We next try to control the coming inflammation to the minimum necessary to the reparative process. I use this language in deference to authority. I do not believe inflammation necessary to repair, for Mr. Paget has shown that it is only in the way; but it is, as far as I know, a constant accident of these wounds, and therefore I am willing to employ the language of the schools. Ice has been employed topically since the last century. Schmucker lauds it extravagantly. Guthrie uses it everywhere. The French surgeons generally have adopted it, but Vidal says, as a general rule, it is a bad practice; that it is used to prevent or cut short inflammation. Now, a certain degree of inflammation is necessary in these wounds; the eschar can not be detached except at that price.

Velpeau says the temperature is not equally influenced throughout the limb by ice. The surface may be very cold, and the *trajet* of the ball very hot. Then we will have an unequal inflammatory action evidently less favorable than if uniform throughout. We have thus a bastard inflammation—a sanious, badly elaborated pus, and wound that progresses slowly toward cicatrization. If there are flaps, or already embarrassed circulation, ice favors gangrene.

Velpeau had a patient in La Charite, who had been treated with ice for thirty days in an ambulance, and he found eschars scattered over healthy portions of the skin. He adds: cold topical applications are only suited to cases in which there is violent pain, and a sensation of heat, without swelling or inflammation. Perhaps a little cold might be applied beneficially in hot seasons. Vidal agrees with Velpeau, with regard to ice, but not cold water. Cold water was applied by the Italians, soon after the invention of gunpowder, but it was first subjected to charms and incantations. It was long in the hands of quacks, and although regulars saw it used, they attributed the success to magical and unchristian acts, that no man of any piety would submit to, as it was unauthorized by the church. Ballingall speaks well of it, so long as it is agreeable to the patient. In other cases, warm fomentations, or cataplasms, may be advantageously substituted. Macleod recommends cold applications until inflammation and suppuration are present, then not. Vidal insists that we should not lose sight of the distinction between these two kinds of swelling after gunshot wounds; the one doughy, indolent, cold, with the color but little altered; the other tense and elastic. In the former, sedatives only reduce still more the vital powers already sufficiently suspended by the action of impinging forces. In such cases we must use stimulating and hot applications: if a reaction occurs, we must then employ our antiphlogistics; but generally with these antecedents, poultices and warm fomentations answer best in the consequents. In the second variety, the opposite course should be pursued.

This question of *hot or cold* was debated in the French Academy in 1848. Valette has given us a resume of the opinions of several distinguished surgeons, and appended the result of his own experience in the Crimea. Bègin thinks the tepid applications are the best. Baudens regards ice as a precious means; the wounded are delighted with it, while morbid heat exists. Huguier confines it to wounds, when the whole extent can be subjected to its action, and those in which strangulation is threatened, or burrowing of pus, as in the foot, leg, knee, hand, arm, face, etc. Roux is opposed to them, he says "we can not hinder inflammation, and should not, if we could, as it is contrary to the natural powers."

Amussat has found advantage in replacing cold by warm water. Valette objects to cold water, that where there are many wounded together, an undue dampness is kept up in the wards, very prejudicial to the health of the wounded. He uses simple dressings—cerate and lint—poultices, when pain ensues, and leeches, if inflammation exists. It is absurd to adopt any method exclusively, when we have so many recommended on good authority. We can always command some of them. Poultices may be made of different substances, bay-root mucilage in Florida, the cactus in Mexico, etc.

In cases of extensive crushing or disorganization of a part, no one would use cold applications. Stimulants and hot applications are the proper remedies, but reaction should be watched, and then antiphlogistics, leeches, etc., should be resorted to if necessary. Phlegmonous erysipelas may be treated, as in Gen. Shield's case by yeast poultices and incisions. It is scarcely necessary to warn surgeons against tents, setons, ointments, etc. The burrowing of pus, and collections of it, should be prevented by means of counter openings, when necessary. Proper bandaging will often save the bistoury. Syringe the wound with tepid water, and remove pieces of cloth, clots of blood, and other foreign bodies. The French use one part of perchlor. ferri., to three parts of water, in profuse suppurating wounds. My own experience with this agent, has left a favorable impression. Cod liver oil was used in the Crimea in these cases. The position of the limb should be such as to relax the wounded muscle, and favor the return of blood. It should not be forgotten that, as the result of wounds, limbs may become contracted and require tenotomy.

CHAPTER V.

AMPUTATIONS.

Cases for amputation were better defined formerly, than at present, since excision has come into fashion. Amputation was at first confined to cases of gangrene. Pott extended it to cases in which the patient's life was more hazarded by the attempts to save, than by removing the limb. His doctrine was "better live with three than die with four limbs."

Lacerated wounds, with loss of substance, rupture of blood-vessels and nerves, extensive denudation of bone, may lead to the necessity of amputation. Guthrie has reported a case where the soft parts were carried away from Poupart's ligament to within four inches of the knee, the artery was laid bare for four inches, and yet the patient recovered. Cases of compound comminuted fractures, particularly high up in the thigh, and those involving joints may also demand this operation. In the thigh cases, the prognosis is unfavorable, and there is seldom reaction enough to warrant the operation if near the hip joint. Out of eleven cases of excision of the hip joint for gunshot wounds, only one patient recovered. This was a soldier wounded by a shell, at Sebastopol, the operation was performed by Dr. O'Leary. The head, neck and trochanter, were removed. The result was, the limb became two and a half inches shorter than its fellow, and was capable of bearing some weight; the patient could swing and advance it, but could not bend the knee, rotation was limited and painful. Williamson says that experience in the Crimea clearly proves the superiority of excision of the head of the femur to amputation, and he thinks it will be more frequently employed, with greater attention to the selection of cases. Accidental recovery of one, does not justify this remark. My own experience does not encourage much hope in these cases.

As to amputation at the joint, Larrey gives us seven cases, he says two recovered and were seen in Poland. Guthrie says they never reached France; he claims that one of his survived, and was the first and only patient seen alive in London or Paris, all his others died.

Fractures may be complicated with wounds of arteries, either at the time or after the fracture. Seeking both ends of an artery, in an unsound part, causes too much mischief. Wounds of the knee joint, with fracture of bones, require immediate amputation, unless excision can be substituted, and this is possible when the popliteal artery and nerve are not injured (Guthrie). Excision of the knee joint, is not yet much used in military surgery. It was performed in one case in the Holstein, and one in the Crimean war; both resulted fatally. The operation has been more successful in civil practice. Absolute rest is required, and this can not, as a general rule, be had in war.

Stromeyer was induced to try excision, because amputation of the thigh had been so fatal, being 77 deaths to 51 recoveries. His patient lived three weeks; Esmarch thinks he would have died in eight days, if amputation had been resorted to. I remark, on this case, that the operation was deferred to the fourth day, when fever, inflammation and suppuration had been set up; ball and pieces of the femur were found loose in the joints, and there was great inflammation of the soft parts. The patient died of pyemia. Amputation is the only means of prevention. If the joint is penetrated by the ball, the surgeon should always amputate. The fatality in Stromeyer's cases was due to bad hygiene, removal of men to the rear for amputation, and, from the number of the patients, being obliged to defer the operations more than 24 hours.

Injuries of the patella do not require amputation, as was proved by two of my own cases in the Mexican war. Stromeyer had the case of a Prussian soldier who recovered with anchylosis after comminution of the patella by a bullet, and another case in which a conical bullet split the patella, and lodged part of it in the bone; it was removed by incision. Hennen reports similar cases.

The crushing of the soft parts, with fracture of the bone, without external wound, may result in inflammation and mortification. Severe shell or round-shot wounds generally require amputation, though apparantly unpromising cases, at times, recover. In a case of Howard's, in the Crimea, the shell carried away 3½ inches of the front of the tibia, leaving the posterior part or shell entire; the fragment was removed, and the man recovered. If splintering takes place in the ankle joint, such cases seldom recover without amputation. Guthrie says, that extensive destruction of the soft parts without division of the bone and artery, does not justify amputation; wounds of both, require it, though many recover from one alone.

I do not consider the question settled as to the necessity of amputation in fracture of thigh or leg, from gunshot wounds. A case of mine recovered in the city of Mexico, and another in San Francisco. Baudens insists upon amputation. He says emphatically, and repeats it, "Every fracture of the femur from gunshot, demands immediate amputation." He says, that in 60 cases, all but one were comminuted; 15 were amputated immediately, 13 of whom recovered; of 20 others, secondary operation, 4 only recovered; the other 25 cases in which preservation of the limb was obstinately persisted in, after removal or adjustment of the splinters, all but two died in the course of four months, and their limbs were deformed and useless. Saurel admits all this as to comminuted fractures,but holds that it is a different matter with clear fractures. He insists that the extent and nature of the lesion, should determine the question as in fracture of other bones; that we must consider the height at which the bone is fractured; those fractures being the more serious, the higher the break. Most French surgeons agree that disarticulation should be immediately done when the upper part of the femur is fractured. But when the superior epiphysis is broken, some, Larrey among them, advise preservation when it can be reasonably attempted.

The surgeon should examine for other injuries, as of chest or abdomen, before he performs amputation. A case of shoulder joint at Cherubusco, with canister wound and broken rib, died from that cause. Many of the wounded will not mention this; therefore they should be questioned. Should there be a chance of recovery from them, amputation may improve it.

Is amputation a promising resource?

I think it is; notwithstanding the unfavorable reports of some statisticians. It is true, we find an alarming mortality after amputation in some cases; but we have as encouraging results in others. Velpeau frequently asks, Is death due to amputation, or in spite of it? Burke reports 80 cases of amputation at Bhurtpoor; all recovered in 14 days. Guthrie, 14 shoulder joint, with one death; Larrey, 16, in Egypt, with 2 deaths; and generally, in the French army, one in 10 die after the operation. I had 2 in Mexico, one died from chest wound.

Macleod's statistics refer only to the latter period of the war in the Crimea, and exclude all the unfavorable period.

	DIED.
Thigh—Primary,	62.0
Secondary,	75.0
Average,	64.0
Parisian Hospital (Malgaigne),	73.9
Hotel Dieu in 1830,	81.8
Waterloo,	70.2
India,	48.7
Mexican War,	100.0
Holstein (Stromeyer),	60.0

I amputated 3 thighs in the Mexican war, and all recovered.

Shoulder—Crimea,	33.3
Primary,	20.2
Secondary,	65.0

—from all the campaigns and hospitals in Macleod's table. These ratios of mortality seem so discouraging, that some are ready to proscribe amputation. But what would have been the result without it? Has the experiment ever been tried? Bilguer, surgeon-general in Prussia, forbade amputation in that service, on account of the ill success attending it. At the close of the war in which 6,000 had been wounded, the Prussian surgeons had not amputated a limb. What was the consequence? One half of those who had fracture of the extremities died; one half of the remainder were unfit for employment—11 he reports as surprising cures. Ballingall disputes even these. Macleod's table of all amputations in the Crimea, give a mortality of 33 per cent. Now, looking to the mortality in civil hospitals after similar amputations for injury, we find it exceeding that in the military hospitals. Ballingall remarks upon this, that the civilian goes from good into bad hygienic influences; and the soldier the reverse. The civilian is cachectic from intemperance, from depressed morale, as he has no hope after the accident—goes through a fever attack in hospital. I do not know under what circumstances Ballingall generalizes in this way. A soldier in campaign always has the best air while on duty, if the camp is well policed; if his officers are intelligent, air can be no better in hospital; and bad as the air is in some hospitals, that to which their inmates have been exposed in mines, factories, and overcrowded dwellings, can not have been much better. The fact that the soldier receives a pension and has no family dependent, may have an influence.

We conclude, then, that amputation is the proper resource in such cases as we have endeavored to point out. It does save life, and essentially diminish suffering; and death ensuing can not be attributed to the amputation, but is due to the injury which required the operation. The danger of pyemia is fully as great from the injury as from the amputation, while the danger of hemorrhage, of tetanus, of gangrene, of exhausting suppuration, and the like, are reduced to the minimum by the amputation.

In reference to the *time for operating*, we make three periods, and distinguish the operation accordingly: First, or primary, from the time of the injury to the occurrence of fever or swelling—say, within 48 to 60 hours. Second, or intermediate, during fever and inflammation. Third, or secondary, after fever and constitutional disturbance has set in. There is no point upon which surgeons are more agreed than primary amputation. It is the only operation which Ballingall will sanction on the field. All statistics favor it. The patient is more willing than at a subsequent period. The only objection is collapse. This, when moderate, I have said, is a good anasthetic; if excessive, it demands stimulation and postponement of the operation. We do not know whether reaction will occur; and if death takes place after amputation, it may be attributed to that. Hutchinson denies the possibility of collapse following injury to a degree forbidding amputation. Guthrie has seen necessity for delay to rally a patient. Sir Stephen Hammick, a naval surgeon, advises to "allow patients to recover a little from shock of accident" before amputating. Naval surgeons generally see the wounded at once. There is not much difference, however. I have operated immediately in several instances.

The collapse is in proportion to the injury. At Cerro Gordo, Lt. Davis, of the Rifles, was wounded in the upper third of the thigh; he never rallied. Macleod says there is an interval before collapse comes on—that chloroform precludes all danger of intensifying shock. Edinburgh cases, a few years ago, tell a different story. I would give chloroform after the battle was over—in the hospital, not on the field. Its administration is unnecessary and impracticable in battle. Larrey agrees with Macleod, and says, "It is demonstrated that shock, far from being a contra-indication to primary amputation, should be an additional motive for performing it—that shock subsides instantly after operation—that of three men in whom he amputated both legs at Wagram, the only one who recovered was the first, and that was done a few moments after he was wounded." It may be true that there is a moment of abeyance of shock, but I have not observed it, and I have seen men almost immediately after their injuries; but when collapse is present, I can not yet recommend a disregard of it. If it be present in the extreme and threatening degree, I have attempted to bring about some reaction before operating. Many reasons demand the primary operation, when necessary at all. Removal from field is painful and irritating; the loss of blood perhaps slow, but sure; exhaustion by this, and anxiety as to events, is prevented by operation on the field, Wiseman, Le Deau, and others, all advocate primary operation. But among the French a different opinion sprang up in the last century. After the battle of Fontenoy, the French Academy of Surgery attempted to determine this question, and gave the prize to Faurè, who advocated secondary amputation. Faurè says that of 300 amputations after Fontenoy, only some 30 were successful. Larrey replied to this, that results must have been very different then from what they were at his time, for they saved more than three fourths of their cases, and some had lost both limbs. This he thinks due to the exercise of more judgment in selecting the right time for amputation—to more methodical dressings—to the more simple, speedy, and less painful mode of operation now in use than formerly. Faurè, however, does not proscribe immediate amputation in obvious cases. He advocated it under certain circumstances, because the operation is more successful in cases when patients have been reduced by sickness.

If we look to statistics in civil practice, we shall find that secondary operations have been most successful in some of the French hospitals, but not in the English or Scotch, except at St. Thomas. In this, we have all dying in primary operations for thigh injury, and only 50 per cent. in secondary. Macleod finds an average, however, to be, in these cases, in civil hospitals, 69.6 for primary, and 75.4 for secondary—not a very great difference in favor of either operation. But in amputation for gunshot wounds of the thigh, we have a wide difference in favor of primary—56.5 to 79 per cent. for secondary. An operation on one in vigorous health, is attended with danger peculiar to that condition. John Hunter remarked this. I think that rest and low diet may obviate some of these risks. Macleod says the difficulty is to recognize cases that demand it, and be sure no internal lesion forbids. But he thinks it will save life to operate in all doubtful cases. The statistics of all amputations certainly sustain this advice, 25.22 primary, 45.1 secondary having proved fatal. Exclude fingers and toes, and we have 37.1 primary, and 60.0 secondary, fatal. It has been remarked, " the farther the injury from the body, the less danger from delay." When the thigh is the seat of injury, in my opinion, the *nearer to the body*, the less the danger from delay, for, in amputations in the upper third, we have seen how general is the mortality. In the lower third, 50.0 died; middle, 55.3; upper, 86.8; hip, 100. Macleod never saw a recovery where amputation was certainly in the upper third. French and Russians found them so hopeless that they abandoned the operation, and thought it better to try to save them without. Baudens says the Crimean war shows operations at the knee joint more successful than the thigh. Macleod gives of this, 6 primary, 3 fatal; one secondary and fatal: proportions the same as in the lower third of the thigh. I mention that the older surgeons amputated only for gangrene. There was a dispute about the propriety of spreading gangrene. Ballingall, in favor, speaks cautiously; of 6 cases, one died soon after operation, but without gangrene attacking the stump; another lived 10 or 12 days, and died of internal injury—broken rib and abscess of liver; a third got well; one got well of the other three. In only one case did gangrene attack the stump. A sloughing stump and this form of gangrene are different.

Secondary amputation is sometimes necessary, for secondary hemorrhage ligatures irritate, and do not succeed here. There is constitutional derangement—phlebitis and sloughing of stump. Intermediary operations are seldom successful, though Fauré says they are better than primary. The knee case I quoted from Stromeyer (fatal), was one of this kind, Every pathological consideration is opposed to it, and it should not be resorted to except in very urgent cases. Now as to the place where operations should be performed, I do not know any safer principle than Velpeau's. "It is generally advised to amputate at the articulation, or in the continuity of the bone above it. The accidents which supervene after amputation have been chiefly attributed to the fissures which extend sometimes to the spongy texture of the upper articular extremity of the broken bone." Kerst remarks that the fissure is always made in the direction taken by the projectile, so when wounded from above down, he was successful in operating a few inches above it. Macleod remarked that the bone is always split downward—this is not always true. The amputation should be above the next joint, if the wound in the bone is not more than three inches below it. This is particularly true in reference to the knee and shoulder, for there is great danger of phlebitis if the fissure extends into either of these joints.

Legouest, in a memoir on this subject, strongly opposes amputation, either primary or secondary, and says expectant treatment has saved more than amputation. He especially opposes the immediate operation. In shaft of bone, Baudens regards it as necessary.

Riley, in 1831, asserted that if these cases were not amputated the men invariably died; and that in a careful inspection of the Hotel des Invalides he had been unable to find a single man that had survived a similar injury, nor a thigh stump for a fracture as high as the middle of the femur. Hutin resumed his investigation, and reached a very different result. Among 4373 he found 143 thigh stumps, and 4230 legs; again, 63 cured without amputation of thigh, and 76 of leg. Considering the seat of the fracture, he reached these results: Fractures in the middle of the thigh; 5 amputations, and 20 cured without amputation; below the middle, 16 with, and 19 without; above the middle, none with, and 24 without. I go on with table now as to leg: He found at the middle of leg 12 with, 22 without; above the middle, 6 with, 20 without; below the middle, 64 with, and 34 without—an unfair result, because he does not give us the number of cases lost in the attempt to save the limb. Saurel concludes that we should fall into a grave error, if we amputated all thigh cases, and that we should confine them to cases where it is comminuted, and the preservation of limb impossible. And much more so as to the leg, as less grave than the thigh, especially when only one bone is broken, though these wounds are worse than when in the upper extremity.

The circumstances of the case should govern—if the man can have rest—well; if not, then amputate, in all cases (the leg, if both bones are injured). If extensive splintering exists, amputate anyhow. If you determine not to amputate, remove the spiculæ. Sometimes the wound heals without, they become inclosed in the voluminous callus—still they are foreign bodies, and sooner or later indicate their presence, by acute pain and persistent suppuration.

We pass now to fractures of the upper extremities, and here we find the results of experience altogether different from those of the lower. Mr. Guthrie says the upper extremities should not be amputated for almost any musket wound. If the injury is done by cannon, or shell, with destruction of the soft parts and wound of the artery, he says it is best to amputate. Here he is too fast—a musket ball may cause extensive comminution and splintering into the joint. If a wound of the humerus is limited to the head, exsect; if it extends to the shaft, amputate. Neither operation is always necessary. Guthrie gives several cases where splinters were removed by incision, and recovery followed. We can not resist the preponderance of opinion in favor of preservation. I confess I did not attempt it in the Mexican war, but the Holstein and Crimean wars have occurred since, and I should act differently in another campaign.

Stromeyer says, amputation at the shoulder joint, is only necessary when the ball enters the inner side and injures the vessels and nerves. He says his experience contradicts Larrey's and Guthrie's. That exsection should be limited to the head, and not the shaft of the bone. He says, of 8 left to nature, 5 died; and of 19 resections 7 only died, and these from pyemia, or too late operation. (Five inches of bone once removed.) As to the shaft of the bone, the same rule applies as in the thigh. If the injury of the soft parts is extensive, and the arteries and veins are wounded, then amputate. An artery wounded with the bone, may recover under favorable circumstances, as in a case treated by Dr. Coolidge. We come now to the elbow joint; and here exsection is so encouraging, as to establish it, in my mind, as the plan. Macleod's report is very favorable. Stromeyer reports 40 cases, and only 6 deaths, with greater or less mobility in nearly all his cases. Guthrie says, if the olecranon, or other portion of a single bone is fractured, no operation is immediately necessary; if both bones of a limb are injured, amputation was, but excision is now the rule. Saurel reports two similar cases, anchylosis in both, with discharge of fragments. Query: Which is preferable: operation with fair chance of mobility, or no operation and certain anchylosis?

Amputation of the forearm is rarely required; as the fragments may be easily removed, and the arteries tied. In wounds of the hand, Guthrie says, we should saw through the metacarpal bones, and not open into the wrist, if possible to avoid it, though I acknowledge this does well if we can make sufficient flap to cover it. Stromeyer thinks that wounds of the wrist do not require amputation, unless there is extreme laceration. A case which occurred when the second row of carpus was traversed by a bullet, and yet recovery followed without the least interference with motion of the hand. When cases require active local depletion, use leeches or incisions to relieve tension of fibrous coverings. Removal of fragments of the metacarpal bones in preference to exarticulation, would be now adopted, either as a primary or secondary operation. Amputation of a finger is attended with very little danger. Tetanus has sometimes, though rarely, followed. Stromeyer says there is not the least danger in primary operations, but after forty-eight hours, they may be followed by violent inflammation and obstinate suppuration, and not unfrequently by the stiffness of several fingers, or of the whole hand. We may say generally, that the removal of fragments of bone is now superseding amputation.

It is scarcely necessary to discuss the various modes of performing amputation, in a work of this chararter. I will only say that where there are two bones, as in the leg, I am in favor of the circular. In the thigh or arm, I prefer the flap.

CHAPTER VI.

WOUNDS OF THE CHEST.

Traumatic lesions of the thorax are among the most important that come under the observation of the military surgeon, whether we regard them in relation to the frequency of their occurrence, the importance of the parts exposed to injury, the interesting phenomena attending them, or the mortality resulting from them. In many cases they are almost instantaneously fatal from hemorrhage, or suffocation. A large proportion of the slain upon the battle field perish from penetrating wounds of the thorax. The mortality from such wounds in those brought from the field alive, is very great, whether the cavity is penetrated or not. Guthrie tells us, that after the battle of Toulouse which was fought on the 10th of April 1814, of 106 cases received in the hospital, 35 died between 12th April, and 28th June. From this, we may see how soon the man may die, and how long he may linger, fluctuating between life and death, and then perish. Even this time is by no means the limit of danger. Of the remainder of the 106, 14 were returned to duty, and the remainder, 57, were sent to England, some to die, and some to be pensioned, but very few of the latter were ever fit for service again. During the famous *three days* in Paris, in 1830, of 40 received in the Hotel Dieu where they had immediate attention and every comfort, 20 died; 10 seriously wounded, recovered; 7 more—in 6 of whom the cavity was not punctured—and 3 wounded by small swords only, recovered. We have also the statistics of 420 cases in the Crimea. Of these 118 died, 226 were returned to duty, and 76 were invalided. This includes chest wounds of all kinds; but when we separate the serious cases we find, 16 cases of lesions of the contents of the cavity without an external penetrating wound, of these, 9 died. Of 33 cases of penetrating wounds with the missile lodged, or supposed to be lodged, 31 died. Of all the penetrating wounds, there were 92 cases, and 74 deaths. The mortality of all chest wounds, was 31.50 of officers, and 28.09 of men; of actual lung wound, 69.56 officers, and 80.45 men.

There has prevailed, among surgeons, great difference of opinion as to the mortality from these wounds. Wiseman says, that "almost all gunshot wounds of the lungs are fatal—that many instances may be given, of recovery from gunshot wounds of the breast, but few from those in the lungs." Houston says, "all wounds penetrating the cavity of the thorax, so as to admit air, are not certainly, nor instantaneously fatal, unless the apertures exceed that of the glottis." This is looking plainly to a certain mechanical cause for the death, which, we will find, has very little to do with it. John Bell remarks, that "wounds of substance of the lung are far from being fatal." Hennen says he has seen "many wounds of the thorax, from pike, sabre, and gunshot, do well ultimately." Dr. Gregory also testifies that "out of 26 wounds of the thorax, received at the battle of Quebec, two only were fatal." From a comparison of these statistics and observations, we may learn both, how dangerous it is our duty to pronounce this class of injuries, when we meet with them, and how much we may rely upon the resources of nature and art in the ultimate recovery of very unpromising cases.

Wounds of the chest naturally divide themselves into wounds of the parietes, and wounds of the viscera contained within the cavity. Fraser, the most recent writer on the subject, has made a number of subdivisions, but I consider them unimportant, and shall not here discuss them separately.

Wounds of the parietes of the thorax may be of every form, from an incision or a puncture, involving the integument only, to a gunshot wound penetrating to the pleura, fracturing one or more ribs, or the sternum or clavicle, and wounding an artery as *e. g.*, an intercostal, or the internal mammary. The incised wound is a matter of little consequence, generally, and requires nothing more than the ordinary dressing, with stitches or adhesive plaster, or both.

The other classes of wounds of the parietes are more serious, particularly in regard to their results. We may have a simple contusion of the soft parts without external solution of continuity, and apparently requiring no other treatment than rest, with local application of some form of fomentation—arnica, for example, and yet this may be followed by very serious consequences within the chest. Guthrie remarks, that the most simple of these results are pleuritis and pneumonia, or both, "yet," he continues, "many severe blows are not followed by such serious consequences," and he gives many cases illustrative of this fact. But sometimes from these blows and contusions, we have a tearing of the lung itself, and the case becomes then most serious. When we have wounds, either incised or gunshot, penetrating to the pleura, we are to expect more or less inflammation of that organ, sometimes extending to the lung itself; this, however, does not always occur, but it is the part of prudence to be upon the watch for it.

The most simple form of traumatic injury of the parietes, is a a stab by a sword or knife. There is but little pain, if any, attending such a wound as this, though the patient is frequently very much frightened. His alarm sometimes assumes the appearance of true shock, and may communicate itself to the surgeon. I have seen several instances of this kind among men engaged in election riots and private brawls. In some of these instances, pleuritis succeeded the wound, though I felt sure the pleura was not punctured. I may bave been mistaken, however, the men were of intemperate and irregular habits, and excited by liquor when their wounds were received, and it is possible subsequent symptoms may have been aggravated from those causes. An aid-de-camp of Gen. Scott received a lance wound under the left scapula, in an affair with some Mexican guerrillas. I felt persuaded, in his case, that the thoracic cavity was not opened, though the pleura may have been injured. This officer's life was in great peril for weeks, from relapse of pleuritis, and though now living and well, there are, no doubt, adhesions of the pleura in the part wounded.

Bloody sputa may occur in these cases, in the course of the treatment, but as Hennen remarks, the hemorrhage is only secondary, and is not so active or alarming, as pours out at once, when the lungs are wounded. In gunshot wounds of the parietes, the ball sometimes may carry in before it a fold of the handkerchief or the shirt, and be pulled out with them, and this either with or without having penetrated the cavity. It is well to bear this in mind, as we may suppose the ball to be lodged, and proceed to useless exploration, when the patient, if questioned, might save us this trouble and subsequent mystification.

When the ribs are fractured, we can readily ascertain that fact, by introducing the end of the little finger into the wound. We may look for more serious consequences in these cases, with more present anxiety and collapse, than when the soft parts alone are implicated. The division of an artery will, of course, be made known by the hemorrhage. The treatment of a gunshot wound of the soft parts of the thoracic parietes, will not differ from that I have already indicated to you, while discussing the general subject of the management of fractured ribs and hemorrhage.

Penetrating wounds of the chest are a much more serious matter. Whether the contused viscera are wounded or not, they are always to be looked upon as dangerous, and call for great vigilance and care in their management. Where the viscera are not wounded, we have more pressing symptoms immediately, in the form of shock, anxiety, dyspnœa, and sometimes syncope, we are always to look for pleuritis and its consequences, and frequently pneumonia. When the lungs are wounded, we have, in addition, immediate danger from hemorrhage and suffocation from blood flowing into the air cells, and into the cavity of the thorax. The secondary dangers are also of an aggravated character—violent pleuritis and pneumonia, or rather congestions of the lungs, tedious suppuration, with hectic cough, emaciation, and, when the bones are injured, with exfoliation.

In gunshot wounds, these dangers are liable to be aggravated by the lodgement of extraneous bodies within the cavity, e. g., balls, pieces of clothing, spiculæ of bone, fragments of equipments, etc. These bodies, when lodged in the cavity of the chest, are always liable to excite local inflammation and its consequences, so that the patient can seldom be considered safe while they remain. Hennen tells us, that in deaths from these injuries, he has frequently found pieces of wadding, of clothes, of spiculæ of bones, balls, etc.; and in one instance, a piece of the charpie, used in dressing the wound, either loose in various parts of the lungs or in sacs formed around them. Again, he says, these bodies may be lodged within the cavity or in the lungs, without producing immediate or eventual ill consequences. In those who recovered, however, the offending bodies have been discharged or extracted through the wound, and sometimes even ejected by coughing. Guthrie confirms these observations. He has seen pieces of wadding, of buttons, of bone, and of cloth, coughed up, but never a ball; though, it is said, even this has occurred. After death, he has seen all these things loose in the chest. Balls more frequently become encysted, and remain without exciting inconvenience. A case is recorded of a man carrying a ball in his chest for forty years. It was received at the battle of Waterloo. He died in London a few years ago. Hennen mentions cases in which they have been encysted in the substance of the lungs, and no inconvenience felt from them. Percy mentions instances in which they have been known to roll about upon every motion of the patient. This I doubt. But however that may be, when they do remain, they are generally confined in sacs. Fraser has enumerated a number of cases of this sort—one in the *Lancet* for Jan., 1847,—where a ball had lodged near the surface of the lung for 50 years; one in the Transactions of the Medico-Chirurgical Society, where a piece of iron hoop had remained in the chest 14 years. These cases are remarkable and interesting in showing such surprising tenacity of life under such severe injuries of the thorax. We can not account for such results, especially when we contrast them with the great mortality following even thrusts with a small sword or the smallest pistol ball, implicating the viscera contained in the thorax. Hennen has given a report of a case, in which a man was wounded between the third and fourth ribs of the right side. The only singularity about the case was, the large irregular wound, admitting three fingers. On the fifth day, while turning the man to examine the wound, a tumor was discovered upon the scapula, and upon opening it, supposing it to be the ball, the surgeon extracted the man's breast-plate, doubled up and enclosing the ball. This man was apparently doing well for three weeks, when he got into a violent rage, and tore off the dressings, with the loss of his life for his pains. But the most remarkable case within my recollection is the one reported by Dr. Cooper, of San Francisco, a few years ago. A young man, 25 years of age, by the bursting of an old gun, was wounded in the side by a piece of old iron which had been used as a breech-pin. "It entered the left side fracturing the fourth rib, and remained in the chest until it was extracted seventy-four days afterward. The patient, at that time, was in a state of extreme prostration; purulent matter was discharging through the opening made by the slug; the left lung had lost its function, and the symptoms of suffocation were most alarming." By a bold and very remarkable operation, after a search of three quarters of an hour with a sound, the body was discovered between the descending aorta and the heart. "The sound was held against it until a pair of long lithotomy forceps was thereby conducted to the spot, and the breech-pin seized and extracted. The forceps could not follow the sound, and be sufficiently expanded to seize the metal, without lifting the apex of the heart considerably out of its position." The Doctor remarks, that the patient recovered rapidly after the operation, and appeared to be as well a few months afterward, as he was before he received the injury, though the left breast remained somewhat sunken.

Though, as we have said, we are to consider all penetrating wounds of the chest as very dangerous, still, if the lung is also wounded, the danger is seriously increased. It is a matter of great importance, then, to determine that fact; and this we shall find to be no easy task. One would naturally suppose that if we find a perforation made by a ball upon the surface of the chest, and an exit-hole at an opposite point, that the chest and its corresponding viscera had been traversed; but this is by no means always the case. Hennen says, he has traced a ball making a circuit of the lungs and escaping at a point opposite that of entrance, as if the man had been shot directly across; this also accompanied by bloody sputa, and yet the lung was untouched. Dupuytren asserts almost the same thing. "It happens," says he, "that a ball traverses the chest from side to side, without wounding the lung." Frazer asserts, that even the conical rifle ball may be so deflected that, however specious the appearances, the pleura may not have been entered, and, in many cases, most certainly, the lungs not wounded. The pleura appears to possess a resilient power that is sufficient to deflect the ball. We may note here, however, that though the pleura may not have been entered, still, in some of these cases, the lung may be torn, from the force of the blow, as occurs in other instances of external violence. When a ball traverses the chest, the wound of entrance will be found round, perhaps depressed, discolored, and more or less bloody; the wound of exit will be more of a slit, or a ragged rent, than a circular hole; the alarm is great, vital powers depressed, the wound may or may not bleed externally, or perhaps even internally; the patient may spit more or less blood, the countenance pale, extremities cold, the pulse variable; the symptoms depending upon or modified by the nature and extent of the injury, the temperament of the patient, etc. Guthrie thinks, that when balls run round the thorax without penetrating the cavity, and make their exit at the opposite side, it is the rare exception to the general rule, and depends upon them striking some impenetrable body, such as a piece of money, a button, a rib, or the like. In such cases, the symptoms of penetrating wounds do not occur, or they subside after the first alarm is over, though the various inflammations may, and often do, follow. Fraser remarks, that in penetrating wounds of the chest, when the patient is placed before the surgeon without delay, there is often little or no anxiety, dyspnœa, or other urgent symptoms. This is in strong contrast with the alarming depression we always observe in penetrating wounds of the abdomen. This, as Fraser suggests, is probably due to the ganglionic system being more directly implicated in the latter. A man was wounded on the 18th June; the ball entered between the ninth and tenth ribs of the right side, posteriorly, and came out three inches from the umbilicus on the same side; no lung symptoms supervened. Another man was wounded the same day; the ball entered anteriorly at the fourth right rib, and made its exit at the inferior angle of the right scapula; there was great depression. Ten days afterward, absence of respiratory murmur, and slight dullness upon percussion of the base of the right lung. 8th July, respiratory murmur again heard, and no dullness. In a few days he was returned to duty. Another, in the same battle, received a ball between the sixth and seventh right ribs, which passed out between the ninth and tenth of the same side. Dullness upon percussion, and absence of respiration at the posterior part of the right lung; no fever or lung symptom supervened. On the 8th July, the respiratory murmur had returned, but the dullness upon percussion remained. Another man was wounded on the 8th September, by a grape-shot, which entered at the left loin, passed transversely upward, and made its exit at the eighth left rib. This patient presented no lung symptoms, and his wounds were so nearly healed on the 20th September, that he was sent to his regiment. Mr. Fraser has given us a number of similar cases, but these are sufficient to sustain his remark as to the absence of symptoms in certain cases.

The signs relied on by observers generally, as decisive of lung wound, in addition to depression, etc., are hemoptysis, dyspnœa, collapse of the wounded lung, traumatopnœa, emphysema and pneumothorax.

Guthrie says that bloody expectoration is positive proof that the lung is wounded, though the absence of this symptom does not prove the contrary. Schmucker, Stromeyer and John Bell all consider it a sign of lung wound. The latter says, "if the patient spit blood, I fear a wound of the lung; if he has an emphysema, I am sure of it." Dr. John Thomson says, "that the lungs have been wounded, may be inferred with certainty in every case where a person spits blood immediately or soon after receiving a wound of the chest." Macleod says that "blood by the mouth and blood and air from the wound, are unequivocal proofs that the lungs have been injured." Hennen writes, "to discover whether the wound has injured the lungs or not, is a point which has given to the older surgeons great room for the employment of their ingenuity in devising possible cases, and has occasioned no small waste of time and wax tapers in ascertaining the exit of air through the passage. A practical surgeon will require but little investigation; bloody expectoration *immediately* after receiving the wound, and the terrible symptoms of dyspnœa, sense of stricture and suffocation, insupportable anxiety and faintness, which succeed, soon enough discovers the fact." Fraser, on the other hand, disputes all this, and thinks that spitting of blood may be a very deceptive sign of lung wound. He records that out of 9 fatal cases in which the lungs were wounded, only one had hemoptysis; out of 7 fatal cases in which the lungs were not wounded, 2 had hemoptysis, and out of 12 cases of recovery, 3 had hemoptysis.

I have no doubt that hemoptysis may occur without the ball having entered the lung, from concussion, as before stated; but still there is traumatic lesion of the lung, a tearing of its substance, or a rupture of one or more vessels. It is, then, more a dispute about words than things. In cases of bayonet or sword wounds, and the like, I should look upon the symptoms as sure. That it is absent in many cases of lung wound, there can be no doubt. It is not safe to pronounce that the lung is not implicated, because there is no expectoration of blood.

That dyspnœa should occur in wound of the lung, we might almost assume *a priori*. Nevertheless, standing alone, we can not consider it as indicating this lesion. It may occur from many causes attending wounds of the chest, exclusive of injuries of the lung itself. Fraser remarks, it may be intense from moral causes. It may depend upon collapse of the lung from admission of air into the cavity of the chest; or upon effusion of blood into the chest, though this is not likely to occur very rapidly after wound of parietes only; it may be, too, that the motions of the chest wall in respiration are so painful as seriously to embarrass that function, etc. When an opening is made into the chest of the dead body, the lung, unless prevented by adhesion, collapses; and it was once, and may still be a generally received opinion, that the same phenomenon appears in the living body; this, however, is by no means the fact. Both observation and experience have settled the point. Hennen remarks: "The sinking of the lung is not a uniform consequence of a penetrating wound of the thorax. We have sometimes ocular proof of this, not only by the close contact in which the lungs lie to the wound, discoverable at first sight, but by protrusions that occasionally happen, and which in the hands of older surgeons were removed by the knife, a practice now rejected and gentle pressure substituted." Guthrie says emphatically, that the lung does not collapse from an opening made in the chest in the living body, as it does in the dead, nor does a wound in the chest, when kept open, cause this collapse to the same extent as it is generally supposed to do in the living body. When the lung has been wounded by a ball actually going through its substance, it does not necessarily collapse, and injuries of its surface lead to no such result." Again he says, "the ball in passing through the lung destroys the life of only the part it touches. The wounds being kept covered, it did not and does not usually collapse, or recede from the wall of the chest, but quickly recovers its state of expansion, however impaired it may be at the time of injury." Here is a case from Frazer, showing that the lung may be wounded, and a large opening made into the cavity, and the lung remain uncollapsed. A man was wounded on the 18th June; the ball entered the thorax at and smashed the third left rib, traversed a portion of the lung, passed through the sternum at the junction of the second right costal cartilage, knocked off an inch and a half of the sternum, wounded the lung, laid open the anterior mediastinum, and made its exit at the third right rib. Upon coughing, air passed through the anterior opening, the lung uncollapsed. Another man wounded on the 8th September; the ball entered posteriorly at the fifth left rib close to the spine, and made its exit above the left clavicle. In this case there was no dyspnœa, and after death, the apex of the lung was found much congested, but neither wounded nor collapsed. In an experiment performed at the London Hospital upon a strong, healthy dog, the following phenomena were observed: "The skin having been reflected in the right side, a portion, one inch in diameter, of the intercostal muscles, between the fourth and fifth ribs, and one inch from the sternum, was entirely cut out. The lung did not collapse, and no special dyspnœa ensued. The left side was treated in a similar manner; the lungs collapsed, and considerable dyspnœa supervened. The dog survived 45 minutes; the action of the heart continued after respiration ceased."

There are numerous other experiments and cases upon record, confirming the fact that the pleural cavity may be opened, and the lung remain expanded. It is not necessary to quote them here. Mr. Fraser says the question remains unsettled, whether the pleura pulmonalis, and the pleura costalis in a normal state, are always in immediate contact; and asserts, if they are not, there must be gaseous matter in the pleural cavity. He refers to two experiments of Dr. Halls,' which tend to show the presence of air, and thinks that the reports of many cases of thoracic wound, in which the lungs have marvelously escaped, can only be accounted for by the pleura not being always in contact.

Mr. Quckett, however, at the instance of Mr. Guthrie, performed some experiments upon rabbits, that seemed to establish the fact, that they were always in contact. Nor can I conceive how, under any circumstances, short of considerable collapse of the lung, they could ever be so far separated as to protect the lung from injury, when a bistoury is plunged three inches into the thoracic cavity of a small dog, as Mr. Fraser states occurred in one of his experiments. But I can not help referring here, to a fact observed in one of his experiments, that is exceedingly interesting. A healthy dog having been suitably prepared and placed under the influence of puff ball, a portion of the fifth right rib was dissected out sufficiently to bring the lung into view, carefully avoiding wounding it. The lung was then distinctly seen to contract upon *inspiration*, and to expand upon expiration. Several explanations of this fact have been advanced. Dr. Hall thinks it due where there is an opening on one side only, the force of the blood in the pulmonary circulation dilating the lung.

Hoadley says, "in expiration, the air in the wounded side was condensed, and part of it, instead of going out at the windpipe, forced its way into the lung of the wounded side, and dilated it till the air within came to an equilibrium with the external air which surrounded it; and in inspiration when the air of the lung of the unwounded side, became rarer than the external air, the lung in the wounded side was compressed, and part of the air within it was by the pressure of the external air forced back into the lung of the unwounded side, till the equilibrium was again restored. Dr. Halleday says: "Should, however, the patient, in making an effort to expire, contract the glottis, the air contained in the lung of the sound side, meeting with no resistance, will, by the communication of the branches of the trachea, expand the lung of the wounded side, so as to protrude at the wound." Fraser, while admitting the philosophical ingenuity of this explanation, objects that it does not explain the whole fact, for it requires a "contraction of the glottis," whereas the fact occurs whether there is contraction or not. Fraser himself has given a very good explanation. It is this, that the lungs are compressed, during expiration, by the ribs, through the action of the intercostal muscles; by removing a portion of them on one side, their compressing action is proportionately impaired, while upon the other it remains complete. So long as the sound side acts, and the wounded side offers no opposing force, the lung upon the latter side will necessarily be carried in that direction. Herein, it strikes me, is an explanation of the non collapse in many cases of penetrating wounds of the thorax. When both sides are opened, collapse is pretty sure to occur. In regard to the occurrence or non occurrence of dyspnœa in these cases, we are not yet much enlightened.

If the wound is small, or if it be kept covered, we will not be likely to have much dyspnœa, nor do I think it matters much, as to this, whether the lung is wounded or not. Fraser attributes the dyspnœa to the lung being hindered from any cause from following the chest wall, and says it will be more intense when the action of the thorax is free, and when, from obstruction in the air passages, the air can not reach the air vesicles, so as to expand the lung to the full extent of the thoracic cavity. But when there is an air opening in the chest wall, so that the air can enter the cavity, and the lung is collapsed, there will be no opposition offered by the collapsed lung, and no dyspnœa. As exemplifications of this theory, he adduces the absence of dyspnœa in many cases, while the lung is compressed and bound down to the spine, as by empyreuma, or when solidified, as in pneumonia. Dr. Fraser, however, is in this case, as in several others, inconsistent with himself; as he has shown that the lung does not collapse in many cases of penetrating chest wound, and does follow the chest, and still there is dyspnœa. Again, in cases of chronic compressed lung or solidified lung, the lesion is gradual. I fancy that in the commencement of these cases, there is always dyspnœa, whereas, in wounds, the interruption of the function is sudden. Mr. Fraser's explanation is to me unsatisfactory. The true cause of dyspnœa, in my view, is deficient oxygenation of the blood, be the mechanism what it may. In Fraser's own table, this symptom was present in 3 out of 9 cases of wounded lung; but in all these cases, the congested or almost hepatized condition of the lung, and its engorgement with effused fluid, show that the want of a sufficient quantity of air in the lungs for vital purposes was the cause of dyspnœa. I conclude, then, it is a valuable symptom in the diagnosis, though not of itself sufficient to determine whether the lung is wounded or not.

We come now to notice traumatopnœa, or the passage of air through the wound, as a sign of wound of the lung. This sign has long been considered by the best observers as infallibly indicating a wound of the lung when it exists. Mr. S. Cooper directs us to "make the patient expire strongly; during the succeeding inspiration, cover the wound as completely as possible to prevent the entrance of external air; after once or twice repeating this process, if air continues to be expelled, the lung must be wounded." Dr. Thompson remarks, "It is often difficult to say, in wounds of the chest, whether they penetrate into the sacs of the pleura; but all doubt with regard to this point is removed, the moment we observe air coming out of the wound upon coughing." There are a number of cases recorded by different observers of the recovery from wounds of the lung where the diagnosis was based upon this fact. Yet Dr. Fraser disputes the value of this symptom also, and he adduces the following case and experiment in support of his view: A policeman in London, while guarding a prisoner, was shot in the chest: "the report of his case, shows that blood and air passed through the wound, and there was a little hemoptysis. He died on the second day, and the lung was found not wounded." This report is altogether too meager to found any conclusions on. It does not appear how much air passed through the external wound, nor with what force. When there is an opening in the chest, and air enters through it, if the chest be compressed from any cause, this air will pass out, but with much less force than is observed in traumatopnœa from a wounded lung. The experiment to which Fraser refers, is this: "A dog was placed under the influence of puff-ball; an opening was made into the right pleural cavity, between the third and fourth ribs. The external air passed freely inward upon inspiration, and outward upon expiration. . . . When the dog was examined, the lung was found unwounded." I make the same objection to this experiment that I did to the case. It is evident that if Cooper's plan had been used in the experiment, the deception from the entrance and expulsion of air would have been prevented. Mr. Fraser's object in all this matter seems to me to have been rather to establish a theory than to ascertain facts. He goes on to say that he is of "opinion that when the lung is really wounded, this traumatopnœa must cease;" and assigns some fanciful reasons for the novelty; and then, upon the same page, quotes from the Director General's report, that this symptom was present in 2 out of 12 fatal cases, and one out of 9 cases of recovery; and adds that out of 9 fatal cases observed by himself, in which the lungs *were* wounded, it was present in two. I can not assent to Mr. Fraser's reasoning, but believe with Thompson, that if air is forced out with coughing, the lung is wounded. The lesion may be of such a character that no circulation of air can take place in that lung, and no impulse can be communicated to the air remaining in it upon coughing; so that, although the lung is wounded, this symptom may be wanting. But if the sign is present, the lung is, without doubt, wounded.

Emphysema, though by many considered a sure sign of lung wound, and probably with reason, in a majority of instances, still may occur without lesion of that organ. A case is on record where this symptom determined the diagnosis, and yet after death the lung was found untouched. It was a case of punctured wound, in which a spike had passed through the scapula into the chest. It is not, however, a usual complication of gunshot wounds. In punctured wounds, it is much more frequent. I have seen it in a pistol wound of the lung, but not extending very far over the surface. Guthrie remarks its rare occurrence. He says a slanting pistol ball may cause it; but it is seen more frequently after long and tortuous wounds made by sword or lance, and occurs soon after the injury. Stromeyer explains these circumstances thus: "A ball passing into the substance of the lung bruises it, and causes an immediate extravasation of blood in the lung substance, so that no air can pass from the air vessels or small tubes into the pleural cavity." Emphysema, when it does occur, and particularly in conjunction with any of the other signs noted, I think may be safely considered as indicating that the lung is wounded. Most writers, in noticing this phenomenon, allude to its trifling character and influence upon the result of the case. It very rarely extends more than a few inches from the margin of the wound, and if it does, may be readily remedied by incisions or enlarging the wound. Hennen, however, mentions a case in which all distinction of chin, neck and chest was obliterated, and the air had even penetrated the cellular tissue enveloping the viscera. In cases approaching this in severity, it must become a formidable disease, and would require few incisions to let out the air, as recommended by Wiseman, Williams, Hunter, Guthrie, and others.

I have now gone over the signs of wound of the lung, and, I think, fairly examined Mr. Fraser's exceptions to the generally received views of surgeons upon this point. I think his treatise calculated to do injury in unexperienced hands, by unsettling their opinions in very plain cases, thus leading to indecision in practice, and uncertainty in diagnosis. He himself admits that, "although he would not place implicit reliance upon any one of the heretofore accepted signs of lung wound, if there were three or more of them present, he should consider their concurrence as strong, presumptive proof of lung wound. To these add, a weak pulse, a cold and clammy skin, and orthopnœa, with effusion of blood, and the presence of the ecchymosis of blood in the loins, and with all these, or a majority of them, it may be considered as nearly certain that the substance of the lung has been wounded, and the danger imminent." With regard to the lumbar ecchymosis, I may remark, that it was first suggested by Valentine, as a sign of effusion of blood into the pleural cavity; that Larrey considers it a pathognomonic sign of this condition, and that Guthrie has seen one case confirming it. I have never noticed it, though I have seen several cases of pleural effusion. It may have existed, however, without attracting my attention.

We come now to the treatment of these wounds. I have already referred to the treatment of wounds of the parietes, and will now take up the penetrating wounds.

In incised wounds, penetrating the cavity, without wounding the lung, the wound should be immediately closed by suture, and the patient directed to keep perfectly quiet. We may look for some pleuritis in these cases as a general rule. Sometimes it is severe, and attended with effusion, etc. We must try to prevent this. If it does occur, it demands its appropriate treatment, of which we will treat hereafter. Mr. Guthrie's procedure in regard to these cases is marked by his usual good sense, and we can not do better than adopt them. He directs the patient to lie upon the wounded part, as a general rule; to allow the pleura of the lung to be applied to the wall of the chest, that adhesion may occur at that point; to cut off the wound from the general cavity of the pleura. But after it is shown that adhesion has not taken place, position is not of so much consequence. He enjoins absolute rest and quiet. Bleeding is not necessary, in his opinion, in these cases until after inflammation of pleura, or lungs, or both, shall have occurred.

In a large and direct wound *injuring the lung*, two pressing indications will probably present themselves; to relieve the dyspnœa, and to arrest the hemorrhage. You may have here two very different forms of oppressed breathing: one, much slower than natural; the other, very rapid. The former, Mr. Guthrie remarks, indicates affection of the nervous system; the latter, important lesion within the chest. In the former, the patient will require stimulus; the treatment in the latter case requires more extended notice. In penetrating wounds of the chest, both theory and observation teach that the patient breathes easier with the wound closed, because, if left open, in inspiration, air enters the thorax by the wound, rather than the lung by the trachea. Mr. Guthrie says, that if the wound will admit of being closed, the difficulty of breathing diminishes, adhesion may take place, and the inflammatory action within the chest cease. He records a number of cases of sword and sabre wounds, penetrating the chest, when great relief was experienced in breathing by closing the wound, many of them with ultimate recovery. In some of them a reopening became necessary, to discharge effused blood and serum. This is to be looked for in some cases, for if adhesion does not take place, and the pleuritis goes on, effusion is a matter of course, and it may be so extensive as to require a reopening of the wound or paracentesis, and so also of the effusion of blood. When this pleuritic effusion occurs after a penetrating injury, it is usually from the 3d to the 7th or 9th day. Mr. Guthrie remarks, that it sometimes takes place in from 24 to 48 hours, and is the evil which in penetrating wounds is most to be feared. When the external wound is so much closed as not to admit of its evacuation, it is commonly the immediate cause of the death of the patient. I doubt this very much, but still, when the dyspnœa is oppressive from the quantity of effused fluid within the chest, there can be no doubt about the propriety of an operation for its evacuation. Military surgeons usually select the site of the wound for this purpose, that is, the wound is reopened. But the point of election may be selected for this purpose. This, as you know, is between the 5th and 6th ribs, one third the distance from the spinous processes of the vertabræ. Should there be a protrusion of the intercostal spaces, it may be a rib or two, lower down. The object is to avoid the diaphragm. Freteau penetrated in dead bodies, between the 10th and 11th ribs, on the left side, and the 9th and 10th on the right side, and always opened into the chest. This is an important point, as it is an operation which is sometimes required for the removal of balls from the chest. They usually gravitate to the angle formed by the rib, the diaphragm, and the spine. We wish then, to make an opening as near its locality as possible. In this connection, Freteau's experiments are important. Baudens says, he has frequently performed the operation with success, in the 9th and 10th intercostal spaces, by making an incision three fingers distance from the spine. Mr. Guthrie has given minute directions for the performance of this operation, in the last edition of his work, to which I would refer the reader. He proposes this operation as well in certain cases of empyema, as for the removal of balls. In cases where a fluctuating external swelling exists, the puncture will be made into that swelling—this is called the operation of necessity.

As to the arrest of hemorrhage, it is plain, that if it proceeds from wounded vessels in the lungs, they can not be reached for any operative procedure, and as the patient's life depends upon its suppression, it will be best in this case also, to close the wound, to allow the lung to be mechanically compressed. Unfortunately in such severe hemorrhages, it is seldom we have a chance of doing anything. But sometimes syncope occurs, and the effused blood then has a chance of coagulating. Close the wound then for the present, but watch for the dyspnœa that will occur afterward, together with more or less effusion of serum, say in three or four days, and then, if necessary, operate for their discharge. But here we must also resort to the other therapeutic means, for the arrest of hemorrhage, as in ordinary hemoptysis—bleeding, the use of acetate of lead, turpentine. ergotine, cold externally applied, etc., means too well known in the profession, to need any extended treatment here.

But if the hemorrhage proceeds from a wounded intercostal, what is to be done? If the wound is more than half way to the anterior aspect of the chest, I doubt whether much bleeding is to be expected from these vessels, particularly if completely divided. But in case they should bleed, the vessel must be secured by some means. Plenck carried a needle round the rib and put a tent under it, to compress the vessel. Theden tried this plan, but unsuccessfully. He then cut the vertebral side of it with agaric. Geran recommends a needle to be passed by the wound and over the upper edge of the rib; to the silk, he attaches a dossil of lint, and draws it over the wounded vessel, then by tying it tightly, the bleeding is suppressed.

Hemorrhage from this cause, however, is very rare. Hennen says he never saw a case.

The next point to be attended to is the removal of foreign bodies in gunshot wounds. Upon the necessity of this, all authors of experience strenuously insist.

When a ball strikes the center of a rib, or passes into or through the chest, the bone is broken into several splinters, some of which are driven in or even carried into the lung, together with wadding, pieces of clothing, etc.; these should be extracted if possible, and the sharp edges of the rib, should be rounded off. Irritation of the pleura or lung and emphysema may perhaps be prevented by this means. Mr. Guthrie most judiciously urges thorough exploration for spiculæ of bone, pieces of clothing, etc. Mr. Fraser directs a careful exploration to be made, to detect suspected foreign bodies, "but the less probing and poking about, the better, unless obvious reasons demand manual interference." "As far as regards the probable presence of splinters of bone, we may be sometimes guided by observing whether the ball passed through the cartilage, or the solid osseous portion of the rib or ribs; in the latter, the presence of splinters is more to be apprehended than in the former case." When a ball strikes a cartilage, we may, of course, be relieved as to the presence of splinters of bone but not as to the ball, pieces of clothing, etc. In these cases, the cartilage is bent inward, and may be replaced by the finger, an elevator, or a bent probe. Mr. Fraser thinks that more damage may be done by poking about the chest in search of foreign bodies, than the advantages that may be gained by their detection may warrant. This may be true, if we use improper instruments; but no one I suppose, would thrust a sharp probe into the chest of a wounded man to detect a splinter of bone or a ball. The finger is the best probe, and if there be reason to suspect the presence of these foreign bodies, and the wound is too small to admit the point of the finger, it may be enlarged sufficiently for that purpose. Mr. Guthrie very cautiously advises that this dilatation should be no larger than is necesssry, but that pieces of shell or of broken lances or swords, require larger incisions. These usually enter through the muscles of the back. When a ball sticks between two ribs, great care is necessary in its extraction; the attempt should be made during inspiration, when the lower rib should be depressed, and elevator passed under the lower edge of the ball, to dislodge it.

Sometimes a ball may be lodged in the sternum; this is one of those bones whose structure admits of a ball being firmly lodged in it. In such a case, the trephine may be necessary for the removal of the ball.

Broken ribs, from gunshot wounds, sometimes gives rise to persistent inflammations and empyema, and require the wound to be enlarged to let out the matter, pieces of bone, clothing, etc. Guthrie gives several cases of this sort. Unfortunately, these patients almost always die from repeated attacks of pneumonia, hectic suppuration, and exhaustion. The best means of guarding against these results is to pick away carefully the broken pieces of bone, to pare off the ragged edges of the rib, to apply proper bandages to the fracture, and to keep the patient lying on that side. The principles of the treatment of this fracture do not differ from those that govern the rib fracture from any other cause.

The next important feature of these wounds is the pneumonia or pleuritis that is so apt to follow. Traumatic pneumonia runs its course very rapidly. Mr. Guthrie says its first stage lasts from twelve hours to three days; its second from one to three days. Pneumonia differs from idiopathic in being more congestive. Guthrie, Hennen, and others, recommend bleeding freely; this, however, was not successful in the Crimea. Fraser opposes it. It is best to adopt the same treatment as in idiopathic, so thorougly and practically expounded by Bennett, with which, we take it for granted, every medical officer is already acquainted.

CHAPTER VII.

WOUNDS OF THE ABDOMEN.

The importance of recognizing the long established division of these wounds into penetrating and nonpenetrating, will be obvious from the statistics furnished by Mr. Macleod in his history of the Crimean war. Flesh contusions and wounds (simple and severe) of the abdomen, occurred among the privates after April 1, 1855, 101 times, and in 17 of these cases the result was fatal. Of 38 penetrating wounds with lesion of the viscera, there were 36 deaths, while of 65 perforations simply, 60 resulted in death. According to Mr. Guthrie, a ventral rupture never fails to occur in the openings made by a musket ball penetrating into or passing through the cavity. A contusion arising from a severe blow, or a ball striking obliquely against the abdomen, or cuts and stabs involving the muscular and tendinous parts, may give rise to serious consequences. Thus the hollow, or even more solid viscera, may be ruptured and the patient destroyed. A kick from a horse has been known to lacerate the ilium. A case is reported by Mr. Guthrie in which a soldier was struck obliquely by a cannon ball on the right side of the abdomen and back, which ruptured the right kidney, and filled the abdomen with blood. It is from the hemorrhage, and not inflammation, that patients die when the fixed viscera are ruptured by blows from cannon shot, falls, etc. The most serious injuries from contusions may leave no external sign of the severity of the accident. Extensive sloughing of the abdominal walls may follow shell wounds, or other severe contusions. Mr. Macleod saw one case where nearly the whole of the anterior wall of the abdomen was destroyed by the sloughing from a shell wound. An accident apparently severe, however, may be followed by trivial consequences, and *vice versa.* Abscesses, as might be expected, frequently follow from the passage of balls which traverse the abdominal walls without entering the cavity. If they strike obliquely, they may be deflected by the strong aponeurosis of the front of the abdomen, so as in some instances to pass half round the body. Their course may be marked by a line on the skin of a reddish-blue color.

The diagnosis may be further aided by the early subsidence of the constitutional alarm, should it occur at all. Mr. Macleod remarks, that the state of tension, of the wall of the abdomen, at the time of the accident, appears to exercise no little influence on the effects produced. When a man, for instance, is lying on the ground, and the muscles are completely relaxed, then the injury inflicted on the contained viscera may be very severe; but if the muscles are in action and tense, then the force of the blow will be somewhat mitigated. It is only in this manner, he adds, that he could explain several anomolous cases that fell under his notice.

The surgeon will often find it difficult to determine whether a ball has perforated the abdomen or not. Mr. Macleod has reported the following case: A ball struck a French soldier just above the crest of the ilium, and about four inches from the spine. It escaped close below the inner end of the clavicle on the same side. At the time he was struck, he was on his knees, being in the act of rising from the ground, on which he had been lying. He had hiccough and considerable prostration for three days, and also an attack of pleurisy, all of which he had recovered from a fortnight after injury, when Mr. Macleod first saw him. Although in this case the ball appeared not only to have perforated both the abdomen and chest, and the diaphragm, yet as Mr. Macleod very properly remarks, it probably ran merely under the integuments, perhaps traversing the diaphragm close to its anterior border, and wounding none of the abdominal or thoracic viscera. As a general rule, wounds which penetrate the abdominal walls, are followed by a protrusion of the contents of the cavity, which are liable to become inflamed, strangulated, and gangrenous, as in hernia. As is well known, sharp instruments frequently pass into the cavity of the abdomen for a considerable distance, without injuring the viscera, which are pushed aside. That a blunt instrument, says Mr. Guthrie, like the small end of a ramrod, should be forced between the loose viscera of the abdomen, without wounding any of them, may be easily conceived; but that balls or sharp pointed swords should do so, is not to be understood so easily. Although such cases have been reported, they must be considered as exceptions to a general rule. In some instances balls, having penetrated the cavity, have passed round its internal contour, and have subsequently made their exit at a distant point, or remained lodged within the belly, whence they have afterward been discharged by abscess, or by the natural outlets. The difficulty in forming a correct diagnosis in some of these cases, may be inferred from the following, quoted by Mr. Macleod. Private P. M. was shot through the abdomen at Ferozeshah. Very slight symptoms followed, so that it was supposed the ball had coursed round the cavity, and had not penetrated. He mentioned having passed some blood in his stools after receiving the wound. The ball had escaped near the spine, having entered in front. He recovered slowly, but perfectly, except that he continued subject to bowel complaints, and finally died of spasmodic cholera, a considerable time after being wounded. At the autopsy, a cicatrix of a gunshot wound was found in the left linea semilunaris, about four inches above the crest of the ilium; and on the same plane posteriorly, another cicatrix, an inch to the left of the spine. The omentum firmly adhered to the internal surface of the anterior cicatrix, and was gathered into a fold or knot at that point. The fold of the intestine, immediately opposite to the cicatrix, presented a line of contraction, as if a ligature had been placed tightly round the gut. The fold of intestine just above this, presented the same appearance, and on the first fold, four inches from the first noticed contraction, and in a line below the umbilicus, was another similar appearance. There was no ulceration of the large intestine, although the upper part of the colon was attenuated, and contracted *in situ*. All these appearances, it will be remembered, from a wound when it was supposed the ball had coursed round the cavity, and had not penetrated.

Mr. Williamson, in his Notes on the Wounded from the Mutiny in India, p. 43, notices the curious fact, that on making a post mortem examination of a case of direct gunshot perforation of the abdomen, the intestine is found wounded in many places, considerably removed from the direct course of the ball. He asks, is this removal of wounded portions of intestine from the line of the ball, due solely to the natural peristaltic action, or to something more than this, as the result of injury? He thinks the latter influence must be considerable, as it has been noticed that under perforation of the intestines by ulceration, there is not only contraction in caliber, but marked *shortening* of the intestinal canal. This action beyond the peristaltic, he adds, may be expected, and really appears to follow equally perforations by injury and disease, thus explaining the withdrawal of the wounded points of intestine from the line of the ball, as indicated by the orifice of entrance and exit.

The symptoms regarded as most reliable in determining the special organ or viscera injured are the position and direction of the wound, the persistent vomiting, the ejection of blood by the mouth or rectum, or with the urine, the escape of special secretions, as bile, by the wound, and the peculiar pain or sensation experienced by the patient. Sir Geo. Ballingall gives the following description of the most prominent symptoms of wounds of the abdominal viscera:—A feeble pulse, great prostration of strength, tension of the abdomen, hiccough, and vomiting. All of these, he admits, may indeed occur in irritable or nervous habits, even when a wound of the abdomen does not penetrate the cavity; but when these symptoms continue for any length of time to harrass the patient, there is too much reason to suppose that the abdomen has been opened. This is rendered certain by the nature of the discharges. In wounds of the stomach, he remarks, hiccough and bloody vomiting are for the most part prominent symptoms; while discharges of blood with the fæces or the urine—both of which are generally voided soon after the infliction of wounds of the abdomen—indicate lesions of the lower intestine, of the kidneys, or of the urinary bladder.

According to Mr. Guthrie, however, when little or no injury has been inflicted on the intestines, the natural and usual action of expelling the contents is generally delayed beyond the time at which, in health, it would in all probability have occurred; and he directs us, should the patient have an inclination to perform this function, to assist by an injection of warm water, or any mild laxative, in order to prevent any unnecessary action of the abdominal muscles, against which the patient must be cautioned. In case of rupture of the intestine in addition to the shock, alarm and anxiety common to wounds of the abdomen, we may expect a rapid swelling and tension of the walls, from the extravasation of gas, or the sudden effusion of its contents.

Wounds of the stomach are not always fatal. A number of cases on record show that patients may recover from formidable wounds of this organ. We can hardly agree, however, with Baron Percy, who, in estimating the fatality of wounds of the stomach, calculates that four or five out of twenty have escaped. Mr. Alcock states, that out of about 3,000 cases of gunshot wounds—(how many of the stomach, he does not mention)—he had seen only one case of recovery where this organ had been penetrated by a musket ball. Mr. Guthrie regards wounds of the stomach as usually fatal, and if the patient escape, it is owing to the fact that the injury is confined to the anterior and upper surface, and does not penetrate both sides.

Wounds of the liver, notwithstanding the great vascularity of this organ, are not necessarily fatal. Those of the gall-bladder have resulted in death at the end of a few days, except in those cases where it had become adherent to the peritoneum from previous inflammation. Mr. Guthrie reports several cases of wounds of the liver, in which the patients recovered. He states that he has never had the opportunity of extracting a ball from the liver during life, although he has seen persons live many weeks, into whose livers balls had penetrated; and he has been acquainted with three persons who had been wounded through the liver, and to whom little subsequent inconvenience was occasioned. Wounds of the spleen are generally fatal. When ruptured by blows upon the abdominal walls from cannon shot, the hemorrhage has filled the cavity and destroyed the patient. Wounds of this organ, from musket balls or from stabs with a bayonet, prove fatal from hemorrhage or inflammation.

Mr. Guthrie has seen two cases of wounds of the kidney, which have led him to believe that they are less fatal than those of the spleen. In one of these cases, which he met after the battle of Waterloo, the ball had passed through the abdomen, entering a little below and to the left of the umbilicus, and coming out behind, nearly opposite and close to the spine. No fæcal matter was discharged from the front wound, but some came through the posterior one, accompanied by a small quantity of urine, indicating a lesion of the kidney or of the ureter at its upper part. The symptoms, at first severe, had subsided under proper treatment, and there was every probability that the sufferer would eventually recover, although Mr. G. was unable to trace the case after the man left Brussels. In another case, abscesses formed over the wounded kidney; the flow of matter was great, and had a urinous smell. The desire to urinate was incessant, but it passed only by drops, and brought the patient "to a state of frenzy;" the discharge from the wounds, which had been diminishing for two days before, suddenly stopped; the pain and pressure became intolerable. He remained at last in a state of the greatest torture for about three minutes, when, during an effort, a burst of urine took place, colored with blood, forcing out with it a hard lump, shaped like a short, thick shrimp, three quarters of an inch long, which proved to be the cloth which had been driven in by the ball. It must have passed from the pelvis of the kidney or the ureter into the bladder. As it was hard and covered by a black crust, it was thought to be a stone when it passed.

Wounds of the kidney are generally complicated with injury of other parts of importance. As Sir George Ballingall remarks, in wounds reaching the kidney anteriorily, by penetrating through the abdomen, we have lesions of the intestine, almost inevitably superadded to the danger from hemorrhage, and extravasation of urine into the cavity of the abdomen. The following case reported by Mr. Guthrie illustrates this observation: Le Capitaine Negre, of the French infantry of the line, was struck on the left side above the hip, at the battle of Albuera, by a musket ball, which went through the upper part of the sigmoid flexure of the colon, and came out behind, injuring apparently the fourth and fifth lumbar vertebræ. As urine came through the opening, the ureter or lower part of the kidney must have been wounded, and as he had lost the use of one leg and much of that of the other, the spinal marrow must have been injured. He was left on the field of battle, supposed to be about to die, and was brought to the village of Valverde three days afterward, in a most distressing state. The inflammatory symptoms had been and were severe; the pain he suffered on any attempt to move him was excessive; the discharge of fæces from the anterior, and of urine from the posterior wound, and by the usual ways, rendered him miserable, and he at last implored Mr. Guthrie to give him the box of opium pills, in order that he might end his misery. He died at the end of ten days, after great sufferings, constantly regretting that the feelings of his attendants, as Christians, caused their prolongation. Such is an example of the terrible nature of a wound of the kidney, through the anterior part of the abdomen. If wounded laterally, or *a posteriore*, if the patient is not destroyed by hemorrhage, he is liable to suffer from extensive and deep suppurations, which, in the end, exhaust him. The surgeon will be led to suspect a wound of the kidney, if there is great pain in the lumbar region, with bloody urine, retraction of the testicle, nausea and vomiting. Sometimes the pain is principally felt in the testis, and the spermatic cord of the side injured.

Wounds of the Bladder.—Dr. John Thomson, in his Report of Observations made in the British Military Hospitals in Belgium, after the Battle of Waterloo, states that he saw no fewer than fourteen cases recovering, in which the bladder had been penetrated by musket balls. In most of these cases, the balls had passed through and out of the pelvis, and the entrance and exit of the ball was generally on opposite sides of the pelvis. In none of these cases, in Dr. Thomson's opinion, had the urine found its way into the cavity of the abdomen. When such an occurrence takes place, the patient generally dies of inflammation within the first week. When the organ has been wounded at the part uncovered by the peritoneum, patients have recovered without unpleasant consequences. In other cases, cystitis has followed with urgent symptoms, requiring the application of leeches, the administration of diluent drinks, and especially opium. We need not refer to the cases in which the ball, when lodged in the bladder, has formed the nucleus of a stone, and has been removed by lithotomy.

In order that the reader may have some idea of the nature of wounds of the bladder, we give the following report from Mr. Macleod, which he regards as a fair example of a penetrating wound: G. private, 57th regiment, was admitted into the general hospital in the summer of 1855. A ball had entered his left hip, close to the tuber ischii, and escaped on the abdomen, two inches above the symphysis, a little to the right of the middle line. Urine escaped by the anterior opening. A catheter was passed into the bladder and retained there. He had no bad symptoms of any kind for twelve days. His urine passed by the catheter, and also by the opening on the abdomen. His pulse remained quiet, and his abdomen without uneasiness. His general health was unimpaired, and his bowels acted regularly. The posterior wound, through which urine never passed, closed rapidly. On the twelfth day, he had severe pain in the abdomen, which was, however, relieved by a dose of opium, and he never afterward had a bad symptom or uneasy feeling, except the irritation occasioned by the urine flowing on the abdomen, which could not be altogether prevented. This urine was loaded with mucus and pus during the period of cure, and he passed several small pieces of bone, both by the urethra, and by the abdominal wound. At the end of six weeks, he could retain his urine, and pass it at pleasure by the natural passage, in a full stream. For a month he had been unable to prevent his urine flowing constantly away. In about two months from the period of his admission, the wound on the abdomen was completely closed by the use of nitrate of silver. Some time afterward this reopened, and he could pass the urine through it in a continuous stream. At length it became permanently closed.

The treatment of wounds of the abdomen, in all their varieties, has been so admirably summed up by Mr. Guthrie that we can render the inexperienced military surgeon no greater service than by giving his *Conclusions*, based upon the most extensive experience.

"1. Severe blows on the abdomen give rise to the absorption of the muscular structures, and the formation, in many instances, of ventral hernia; this may in some measure be prevented during the treatment, by quietude, by the local abstraction of blood, and by the early use of retaining bandages.

2. Abscesses in the muscular wall of the abdomen, from whatever cause they arise, should be opened early; for although the peritoneum is essentially strong by its outer surface, it is but a thin membrane, and should be aided surgically as much as possible.

3. Severe blows, attended by general concussion, frequently give rise to rupture of the solid viscera, such as the liver and the spleen, causing death by hemorrhage. When the hollow viscera are ruptured, such as the intestines or the bladder, death ensues from inflammation.

4. Incised wounds of the wall of the abdomen to any extent, rarely unite so perfectly (except, perhaps, in the linea alba) as not to give rise to ventral protrusions of a greater or less extent.

5. As the muscular parts rarely unite in the first instance after being divided, sutures should never be introduced into these structures.

6. Muscular parts are to be brought into apposition, and so retained principally by position, aided by a continuous suture through the integuments only, together with long strips of adhesive plaster, moderate compression, and sometimes a retaining bandage.

7. Sutures should never be inserted through the whole wall of the abdomen, and their use in muscular parts under any circumstances is forbidden, unless the wound, from its very great extent, can not be otherwise sufficiently approximated to restrain the protrusion of the contents of the cavity; the occurrence of such a case is very rare.

8. Purgatives should be eschewed in the early part of the treatment of penetrating wounds of the abdomen. Enemata are to be preferred.

9. The omentum, when protruded, is to be returned, by enlarging the wound through its aponeurotic parts if necessary, but not through the peritoneum, in preference to allowing it to remain protruded, or to be cut off.

10. A punctured intestine requires no immediate treatment. An intestine when incised to an extent exceeding the third part of an inch should be sewn up by the continuous suture in the manner recommended.

11. The position of the patient should be inclined toward the

wounded side, to allow of the omentum or intestine being closely applied to the cut edges of the peritoneum. Absolute rest, without the slightest motion, should be observed. Food and drink should be restricted, when not entirely forbidden.

12. If the belly swell, and the propriety of allowing extravasated or effused matters to be evacuated seems to be manifest, the continuous suture or stitches should be cut across to a certain extent, for the purpose of giving this relief.

13. If the punctured or incised wound be small, and the extravasation or effusion within the cavity seem to be great, the wound should be carefully enlarged, and the offending matter evacuated.

14. A wound should not be closed until it has ceased to bleed, or until the bleeding vessel has been secured, if it be possible to do so. When it is not possible so to do, the wound should be closed, and the result awaited.

15. A gunshot wound penetrating the cavity can never unite, and must suppurate. If a wounded intestine can be seen or felt, its torn edges may be cut off, and the clean surfaces united by suture. If the wound can neither be seen nor felt, it will be sufficient for the moment to provide for the free discharge of any extravasated or effused matters which may require removal.

16. A dilatation or enlargement of a wound in the abdomen should never take place unless in connection with something within the cavity rendering it necessary.

17. If the epigastric, circumflexa ilii, or other artery in the wall of the abdomen, be injured and bleed, the wound should be enlarged, and the bleeding vessel secured by ligature. If the main trunk or the external iliac artery be sought for and tied, the patient will in all probability die.

18. When balls lodge in the bones of the pelvis, they should be carefully sought for and removed, if it can be done with propriety and safety.

19. In a wound of the bladder, an elastic gum catheter should be kept in it, frequently without a stopper, until the wound is presumed to be healed—unless its presence should prove injurious from excess of irritation, not removed by allowing the urine to pass through it by drops as it is brought into the bladder.

20. In all cases in which a catheter can not be introduced, in consequence of the back part of the urethra or the neck of the bladder being injured, an opening for the discharge of the urine

should be made from the perineum into the bladder. It is essential to life.

21. The treatment of all these injuries must be eminently antiphlogistic, principally depending on general and local blood-letting, absolute rest, abstinence from food, and in some cases almost even from drink, the frequent administration of enemata, the early exhibition of mercury, and especially of opium, in the different ways usually recommended, with reference to the part injured."

CHAPTER VIII.

WOUNDS OF THE HEAD.

Wounds of the head may be divided into those which involve the scalp, and those which implicate the cranium and its contents. Dr. Thompson, in the work already quoted, states, that in his visit to the wounded, after the battle of Waterloo, he found where only the soft parts covering the head had been wounded by the sabre, or by musket balls, the wounds in general healed very readily. He saw very little of the erysipelas which is said to be so common an attendant upon wounds of the head. Mr. Macleod says, that from April 1, 1855, to the end of the Crimean war, the returns show a total of 630 cases of gunshot wounds of the head, attended by contusion merely, more or less severe, and eight deaths are recorded among these cases. Of gunshot fracture without known depression, 61 cases appear, and 23 deaths therefrom. Of cases of fracture and depression, followed by censorial disturbance, 74 cases are mentioned, and 53 deaths therefrom; while of wounds penetrating the cranium, 67 cases, and 67 deaths are recorded. Of 19 cases in which the skull was perforated, all died. The trephine was employed 28 times, and of these cases, 24 ended fatally.

After quoting with approbation the observation of Mr. Guthrie, that injuries of the head, affecting the brain, are difficult of distinction, doubtful in character, treacherous in their course, and, for the most part, fatal in their results, Mr. Macleod adds, "Of all the accidents met with in field practice, these are, beyond doubt, the most serious, both directly and remotely—the most confusing in their manifestations, and least determined in their treatment: there is no accident which the surgeon takes charge of with more fear and hesitation, as in no class of cases does he feel so much the mystery that surrounds and guards our life; for while in some cases death follows the most trivial injury, in others, a vast amount of destruction, and even removal of brain-matter, causes little, if any disturbance."

We find every variety of injuries of the head in war, resulting from musket balls, sword, grape and shell wounds. A ball striking obliquely, and its force nearly spent at the time of contact, may give rise to a mere contusion of the soft parts of the bone. A ball "brushing" over the skull, may rupture the vessels between the skull and dura mater, or open the longitudinal sinus, as occurred in a case in the Crimea. Stromeyer attributes pyemia to the effects of a grazing shot, as it may give rise to inflammation of the bone, and of the veins of the diploe, and pus thus enter the system. A glancing shot may completely destroy the skull without leaving any marks upon the scalp.

At the battle of the Alma, a round shot, "*en ricochet*," struck the scale from an officer's shoulder, and merely grazed his head as it ascended. Death was instantaneous. The scalp was found to be almost uninjured; but so completely smashed was the skull, that its fragments rattled within the scalp as if loose in a bag. Even that fearful missile, the shell, may crush the skull, without opening the scalp, as in the following case reported by Mr. Guthrie: A French grenadier was brought to the field hospital, the second day after the battle of Salamanca, who had received a blow on the left side of the head, probably from a piece of shell, which had caused a contusion and swelling on the left parietal bone, with a graze of the scalp, but without any opening communicating with the bone. This swelling, on examination, was so soft, and the feeling of depressed bone beneath so distinct, combined with the fact of the continued lethargic state of the patient, that Mr. G. did not hesitate to lay it open, when the bone beneath was found broken in several small pieces. On clearing away the blood with which the tumor was filled, two of the pieces, which were loose, were readily raised and removed by the elevator and forceps, and egress given to an ounce or two of blood, which was extravasated beneath, apparently from the rupture of the vessels passing between the dura mater and the bone. The patient regained his senses in the course of the night and morning of the third day, and under a strictly antiphlogistic treatment, gradually recovered, some other small pieces ot bone coming away, and one or two others apparently re-uniting to the uninjured parts, showing, says Mr. G., that it is not always necessary to remove every portion of bone which may be broken, provided any bond of union remains, and especially that which exists between it and the dura mater.

Dr. Thompson remarks that among the wounded at Waterloo, it was found that when the sabre had struck the head perpendicularly, the effects produced were extremely diversified. In some cases, the external table of the cranium was divided, the internal remaining uninjured. In a Frenchman who had received twenty sabre cuts in different parts of the body, and who died from the symptomatic fever appearing to arise from the high degree of inflammation attendant upon a wound of the elbow joint, there were found, on examination after death, not fewer than thirteen cuts of the upper part of the cranium, penetrating only its external table, without any inflammation having been communicated to the brain or its membranes. In other cases where the head had been struck obliquely by the sabre, portions of the cranium had been removed, without the brain appearing to have sustained much injury. Several cases are on record, in which a part of the skull has been sliced away by a sword cut, and yet, after being immediately adjusted, has adhered. Mr. Macleod had under his charge, after the fall of Sebastopol, a Russian soldier who had received such a wound, although, in his case, the bone was not entirely detached. The left parietal was cleft, so as to be almost separated. He would allow no one to touch his wound, except a comrade. His recovery was complete, the brain never showing any tendency to protrude, although visible throughout the whole extent of the wound.

The wounds inflicted by shell are the most terrible seen in war. As illustrative of these injuries, we give one or two cases, as reported by Mr. Macleod. An artilleryman was wounded on the 18th of June, by a piece of shell, over the back part of the head, and rendered insensible. He soon recovered, rose, and walked unassisted to the general hospital. No fracture was at first detected, and the lacerated scalp-wound which existed was dressed simply by the surgeon under whose charge he fell. Headache alone was complained of for some days, during which period he was kept low and freely purged. When the wound was nearly healed, he was unfortunately allowed butcher meat and a gill of rum. About a week afterward, severe cerebral symptoms rapidly and suddenly showed themselves, and the wound took on an unhealthy action. The injury was now more carefully examined, the scalp being incised to assist the investigation. A fracture of the occipital bone was found. Bleeding was encouraged from the incision; leeches were placed on the mastoid processes; he was well purged, and cold applied to the head; his diet was again reduced; the unfavorable symptoms almost immediately subsided, and by the use of low diet and purgatives, soon totally disappeared, never to return. In this case, adds Mr. Macleod, a too generous diet caused the appearance of the unpleasant symptoms which supervened, and which, if not promptly arrested, would have been fatal. The local bleeding, he thinks, assisted materially; but the active purging, the cold applications, and the low diet, were the chief means of saving him.

Mr. Macleod saw one case where the whole frontal bone was driven deeply into the brain by a shell, yet the patient survived twenty-four hours.

We give another case where a private was struck, on the 15th November, by a piece of shell, over the vertex of the head, and felled to the ground. He was found, apparently, dead. The surface of the body was cold, his pupils widely dilated, and insensible to light, and no respiration or circulation could be detected. His face was much scratched and congested. Some blood flowed from the right nostril, and the superficial veins of his neck were gorged. The main wound in the scalp extended nearly from ear to ear, across the vertex; and lesser wounds passed in different directions from this great one. The flaps of the scalp were reflected in various ways. A large portion of the bone was seen to be destroyed, and the space left was filled with coagulated blood. The patient was seen by several surgeons, and so impressed were they that life was extinct, that he was carried to the tent set apart for the dead. Twenty-five minutes afterward, on being again visited, some faint signs of life were observed. There was a flutter at the wrist, and an occasional sigh. Profuse bleeding from the head followed, and on the clot, which was seen to be mixed with cerebral matter, being removed, it was found that the bones forming the vertex were destroyed to the extent of 2¼ to 2½ square inches. The surface of the dura mater was scratched, but not torn, except at one spot—at the lateral and posterior part of the wound—where it was lacerated, and from which a spicula of bone an inch long, and which was imbedded in the right hemisphere of the brain, was removed, a piece of cerebral matter the size of a nut adhering to it.

The brain at this part seemed soft and broken down. Some depressed bone was elevated, and all loose scales removed. The scalp was brought together by suture, and lint wetted in cold water applied. Next day the patient was quite unconscious, lay on his back, and breathed regularly and naturally. His pulse was very weak, and his surface warm and moist. He passed his urine in bed. His pupils were dilated and insensible to light. He could swallow freely. During the two following days, his state was unaltered. Both eyes became affected with strabismus. The treatment consisted of purging, cold to the head, and the most sparing diet. On the fifth day.

there were some signs of returning consciousness. He tried to change his posture, and crossed his arms on his breast. His pupils acted freely, and a profuse perspiration covered the surface of his body. On the following day he again relapsed, and the wound, which had begun to suppurate, now became glazed and dry. When his bowels were made to act freely, he again improved and became conscious. He complained of pain in the head, and down the left side of his body. Thus he went on till the eleventh day, being conscious and able to speak. His bowels were carefully kept acting. His pupils had, up to this time, come to contract and expand freely, and the wound was suppurating kindly. He slept much and expressed a great desire for food. On the eleventh day he became suddenly restless and delirious, particularly at night. The strabismus returned. His eye became dull and semi-glazed, and his pupils were widely dilated and little affected by light. By the eighteenth day, these untoward symptoms had, in a great measure, abated. He was sensible and craved for food. His left side was found to be paralysed, the face, however, not being implicated. His pupils were still somewhat dilated but active. On the twenty-third day his sleep was natural. From that time he continued to improve, except that, if his bowels were for a day unrelieved, the bad symptoms immediately reappeared. He left for England in January, apparently well. In May, however, he was admitted into Fort Pitt, on account of general loss of sensibility and motion, partial in the upper, but most complete in the lower extremities. In June he could draw up his legs and stretch them out in bed.

Mr. Macleod, in commenting upon this very interesting case, remarks that the intermittent headaches spoken of in this report are among the most troublesome sequences of injuries of the head, and that the remedies which seemed to him of most service, were blisters to the nape of the neck, morphia, and a careful regulation of the bowels and diet.

Military surgeons have long noticed the difference of character between a fracture of the cranium produced by balls, and those commonly met with in civil practice. The concentration of its force on a small point, the greater support afforded to the outer than the inner table, and the diminished force of the ball as it passes through each, causes a splintering of the inner table, and a laceration of the brain and its membranes. Mr. Macleod is inclined to believe that the character of the fracture in the skull produced by the large conical, is considerably different from that occasioned by the round ball.

The destruction by them of the outer table, always appeared to him much greater than by the round ball, thus rendering the size of the openings in the two tables more nearly equal than after a wound by the latter. On this account, he thinks the true punctured fracture is less seen now in military practice than formerly, although he admits it requires a larger number of observations than he possesses to substantiate this opinion. The round ball has been known to penetrate the outer, without injuring the inner table of the skull, but the conical ball, says Mr. Macleod, not only penetrates, but perforates, and almost always proves fatal. A musket ball may give rise to a fracture of the inner, without that of the outer table. Mr. Williamson has reported a case of this kind, which proved fatal from compression of the cerebral substance by coagulated blood. The ball was a conical one, which, says Mr. W., would have led one to expect quite the opposite injury. He thinks it probable that other cases of this kind have occurred, and have not been detected on post-mortem examination, for in the instance to which he refers, the fissure was not detected until the calvarium was macerated. As the case is an instructive one, we give it in full. Considered in connection with the terrible case of fracture from shell, and recovery, which we copied from Mr. Macleod, it forcibly illustrates the truth of Mr. Liston's aphorism that "no injury of the head is too slight to be despised, or too severe to be despaired of." Private J. Burke, 55th regiment, aged 19, walked home from the trenches, and was admitted into hospital, August 24, 1855. He said that when at the rear, a musket ball, which he found afterward, struck him on the head. On examination, a distinct linear slit, about three inches long, and running parallel with the axis of the brain, was observed situated over the upper surface of the right parietal bone. On introducing the finger, the bone was found quite bare, but no fracture or depression could be discovered. There were no general symptoms of disease of the head. The head was ordered to be shaved, and cold water dressing applied. August 29; this evening the whole scalp was observed to be swollen, but not at all reddened. The œdema was greatest on the right side of the head and face. The edges of the wound looked unhealthy and green, and there was a peculiar smell from it. He complained of a want of power in his left arm; the muscles of the face were slightly twisted toward the right side; he could move his legs freely; a crucial incision was made through the wound, the flaps retracted, and the bone carefully examined. No injury of its intimate structure could be detected, but a distinct black line marked the course of the ball; the pulse was small and weak. Numerous free incisions were made here and there over the swollen scalp; and from these wounds a great deal of serum escaped. On the 30th August, the symptoms of hemiplegia were more distinct; the œdema of the scalp quite gone, and the scalp looked more healthy. The bone appeared dead. September 5th, he had one slight convulsion in the morning, and his respiration was more hurried. At a consultation held, no operation was deemed advisable. He had been put under the influence of mercurials. September 6th, he was much weaker; his respiration more hurried; he had another convulsion, and died comatose in the evening. Mr. W. thinks that the compression in this case could not have been relieved by trephining, as it was caused by coagulated blood; and secondly, if it had been performed, and the dura mater punctured when it was in a state of inflammation, the chances of a fatal issue would have been greatly increased.

Dr. Thomson, in his report, states that among the wounded at Waterloo he saw enough to convince him that the separation of the tables of the skull, and the lodgment of balls between them, is by no means an unfrequent occurrence. This has been observed most frequently at the fore part of the head. Sometimes the ball, by striking the head obliquely, or impigning against one of its angles, is split, one half flying off, the other lodging between the tables of the skull. One of the most remarkable circumstances, says Mr. Macleod, connected with gunshot wounds of the head is, that they are not more universally followed by concussion, or that the symptoms of concussion, when produced, are often so temporary in duration. Men have frequently told him, after receiving wounds of considerable severity, that they experienced merely feelings of passing "weakness" when struck.

As to the danger from wounds of the head, Mr. M. regards it as established that those of the side of the head are attended with the most risk, and that a descending scale will give the following order: the fore part, the vertex, and the upper part of the occipital region; the last being decidedly the least dangerous. He admits, however, that remarkable exceptions to this graduating scale do occur. Age, also, modifies the effects of injuries of the head, and, according to Mr. Guthrie, the wonderful escapes and successful operations on the head, have been, in general, below puberty.

It was the opinion of Hennen, that one half of the injuries of the head are left dead on the field, or die before assistance can be afforded. Indeed, if we are to credit writers on military surgery, it would seem that surgical interference in many cases of gunshot wounds of the head has been of injury rather than of benefit to the patient. Many have recovered under circumstances which forbade any attention being paid to them, and Mr. Macleod declares that these happy results were the more marked when privation was added to this neglect. He adds that Larrey, Guthrie, Ballingall, and the Indian reports, all confirm the observation long ago recorded by Dease, that "those patients who neglected all precepts, and lived as they pleased, did just as well as those who received the utmost attention." At this we need not wonder, says Macleod, when we remember in what the "utmost attention" consisted, viz.: the probings, pickings and trephinings which form the more orthodox and approved practice. To use the language of John Bell, when describing the practice of the ancients, we may say of those who adopt this meddlesome interference, we are to believe that every capillary fissure is attended with peculiar danger, and that without the most adventurous operations the patient can not live. Name me, says Mr. Bell, one absurd or cruel measure—the amputation of large pieces of the scalp—the widening of fissures—the perforating the cranium with many trepans—and opening the dura mater for every idle suspicion or imaginary purpose—name me any extravagance for which their works do not afford us a precedent. Very recent writers inculcate the doctrine that we should seldom or never have recourse to the trephine. To apply to them the language which John Bell employed in reference to those he called modern authors, they would persuade us that the more violent the fracture the less the danger; that our patient, though he lie in a deadly stupor with fracture of the skull, or deep wounds of the brain, needs but to lie undisturbed or unassisted to insure his perfect recovery.

The advocates of each of these extreme opinions can bring forward cases corroborating their position. They can, on the one side, refer us to instances like the one reported by Schmucker, where the trephine was applied eleven times in less than a month, and so little was the patient inconvenienced by the operation that he seldom went to bed after it, and once he actually went to market within an hour after its performance. We might refer to other surgeons who, as Sir Geo. Ballingall expresses it, practiced with unrelenting perseverance the perforation of the skull, as if to show how much additional injury the cranium and its contents could sustain, and to prove that the means adopted to protect the brain from external injury are alto-

9

gether superfluous. But this is surely unnecessary. Nor need we dwell upon those exceptional cases, where patients have survived extensive mutilations without the use of the trephine, offered by those who adhere to the expectant treatment. There can be no question that the restriction which has been placed on the use of the trephine, is a great improvement on surgery; but when we reflect upon the numerous cases in which we have been consulted, where the remote effects of depressed bone have been manifested in epilepsy, idiocy, impaired intellect, and cerebral derangement of various kinds, we are forced to conclude that more reliance has been placed upon the expectant treatment than it deserves. This accords with the observation of Mr. Guthrie. "A patient very often survives a mere depression of the skull; he may, and occasionally does survive a greater depression of the inner than of the outer table; but I do not believe that he ever does survive and remain in tolerable health, after a depression with fracture of the inner table, when portions of it have been driven into the dura mater. If cases could be advanced of complete recovery after such injuries, I should not consider them as superseding the practice recommended, unless they were so numerous as to establish the fact that wounds of the dura mater and brain by pieces of bone, are not extremely dangerous." At another place he states, that the result of his experience has rendered it imperative in his mind to remove at once all portions of bone or foreign substances which may have, or may be supposed to have penetrated the dura mater in adults, although no symptoms of compression should be observed. If the wound in the dura mater should not be sufficiently large to allow the offending body to be extracted through it, the opening must be increased to enable it to be withdrawn without further laceration, and all substances which are irritating, or are likely to irritate the brain, should be removed at once, unless the attempt should give rise to great suffering, or convulsions be present, or great difficulty is encountered in seizing the extraneous body. As an illustration of the difficulty experienced in some instances, we quote the case of Mr. Brougham, related by Sir Philip Crampton. Mr. B.'s gun was accidentally discharged, and fractured the upper part of os frontis in small pieces, and drove the greater number of them deep into the substance of the brain. On attempting to remove one large fragment, on the second day, which was buried in the brain, the whole body was shaken by a convulsive movement, and the patient moaned deeply. Sir P. desisted from all further attempts to extract the splinters, and as even washing the parts gave rise to a sensation which the patient described as dreadful, he desisted from that also. The discharge contained a large proportion of softened brain, mixed with blood, but the wound itself was not so much as washed for twenty-two days, and even then nothing more was done than to lift off the small fragments of bone as they became detached by the efforts of nature. This patient recovered. The practice adopted in this case is supported by the high authority of Mr. Colles, who advises the surgeon to defer the extraction of the fragments for a few days, to give time for the adhesive inflammation to take place, which, he says, hardens the part of the brain involved, circumscribes the depressed piece, and thus enables us more readily to lay hold of the fragment of bone. Mr. Guthrie, however, condemns this delay, believing that the patient has a much better chance of escaping cerebral irritation, inflammation, and suppuration, as well as hernia cerebri, "and all other evil," where the local and the general treatment are alike immediately decided and efficient. He gives us the details of a case which he saw at Antwerp, and in which he gave his opinion, "without hesitation," that the bone and ball ought to have been removed in the first instance, when he would have had a better chance for his recovery. The operation when afterward performed for the removal of the loose pieces of bone, he thinks, placed his life in great jeopardy. He reports the case as illustrative of many important points, and on this account we reproduce it here:

William Rogers, aged 19, of the 32d regiment, was wounded on the 16th of June, by a musket ball, which entered at the inferior angle of the left parietal bone; it knocked him down, and for a few minutes rendered him senseless. On recovering his mental powers which he soon did, he found that he was unable to speak, not so much (as he says himself), from the want of power to form words, as from the incapacity of giving them sound. He was conscious of everything passing around him, and reasoned correctly; he retired out of the reach of shot, and then lay down for the night. On the following morning, finding the pickets retreating, he fell back himself on Brussels, where he was examined and dressed. On the morning of the 18th, he reached Antwerp on horseback, very giddy, and overwhelmed with fatigue, fasting and watching; he was admitted into the Minime General Hospital, and put to bed, when he soon fell into a sound sleep, which with some tea, refreshed him much. On examining the wound, June 19th, the ball was found to have passed obliquely upward and backward at least two inches, and could be distinctly felt with a probe. It gave more the idea of having raised the outer table, than that of having depressed the inner; both tables must, however, have been displaced. The defect in speech, was in some measure restored, and this, with giddiness, were the only symptoms of compression. A poultice was placed over the wound, a sharp purgative given, and spoon diet ordered. On the 20th, the pain and giddiness having increased, with annoyance from noise and exposure to light, twenty-six ounces of blood were taken from the arm. The following day, the purgative was repeated, and the patient was much relieved; a faltering in the speech continued for many days. Everything went on well, the wound was nearly healed, and he was considered almost fit to be discharged, when, on the 16th of July, the wound began to open; on the 18th, it was dilated, and a portion of the cranium removed by the forceps, which was soon followed by symptoms of inflammation of the brain, and twenty ounces of blood were taken immediately from the arm; purgatives and diaphoretics were ordered, and the strictest abstinence enjoined. Venesection was repeated on the 23d, as well as the other means usually adopted to reduce high action. 24th, completely relieved. Saline mixture continued; a little meat soup allowed. 26th, another portion of the cranium removed, the dura mater being fully exposed; the general health in the best state. August 3d, doing remarkably well; the wound healthy; the pulsation of the brain evident; the power of speech perfectly restored. The ball yet remains in, according to the opinion of the patient (a fine intelligent lad), and, he thinks, has gradually descended towards the petrous portion of the left temporal bone. He was discharged the service, and sent to England at the end of the month—"well." The ball was still lodged, however, and Mr. Guthrie thinks it more than probable that he did not long survive, which, he adds, he might have done, if the ball had been removed when it was first felt within the skull.

He thinks the following case, from the Baron Larrey, may be advantageously read in connection with the one just related: An officer was wounded on the right side of the forehead by the point of a lance, which passed upward, making a deep groove in the frontal bone. On the tenth day he was attacked by tetanic symptoms, with loss of sight of the right eye, and convulsive movements of the lid. The external parts were all now divided with the greatest benefit, the tetanic symptoms subsiding within twenty-four hours. On the twenty-fifth day, symptoms of inflammation and of effusion on the brain supervened, and he died on the twenty-seventh day after the receipt of the wound. On opening the head, a portion of the inner table was found detached, and the anterior lobe of the brain in a state of suppuration. Larrey adds: "I had in this case to regret that I did not apply the trephine, occasio prœceps, judicium difficile."

In reference to a question upon which so may opinions prevail, it can not be without interest to know what an authority like Sir Geo. Ballingall has advanced: "In such cases, when the fracture is simple, the general rule is not to perform an operation for elevating the bone, unless the presence of urgent symptoms demands it.

In cases of compound fracture, on the contrary, with any considerable depression, it is advisable to elevate the bone immediately, as a likely means of relieving the brain, and obviating, not only present evils, but future bad consequences. This is the rule which appears to me most consonant to the dictates of common sense: it is the practical rule inculcated by Sir Astley Cooper's extended experience, and it is the conclusion come to by Sir Benjamin Brodie, contrary to his original prepossessions, and after comparing deliberately a great number of cases bearing upon this point."

Having presented to the reader the views of the distinguished authors just quoted, it is proper that, in conclusion, we should also furnish them with those of two of the most recent writers on military surgery, viz: Dr. Stromeyer, of Hanover, and Mr. Macleod, to whose Notes on the Surgery of the Crimean War we have had occasion so frequently to refer. For our knowledge of Dr. Stromeyer's opinions we are indebted to an extended analysis of the work in the British and Foreign Medico-Chirurgical Review, Jan., 1856. Dr. S. states, after the battle of Kolding, in Schleswig, April 23d, 1849, there were eight gunshot fractures of the skull, with depression, and more or less considerable brain symptoms, in the hospitals at Kolding, Christiansfelde, and Hadersleben. With but one exception, the detachment of the fragments in these cases was left to nature. All recovered; but the one from whom some fragments were removed on the 7th day, it is reported, was placed in considerable danger "by this treatment." All of the patients, Dr. S. believes, were saved by simple antiphlogistic measures. From the two campaigns of 1849 and 1850, Dr. S. possesses the notes of forty-one gunshot fractures of the skull, with depression. There was no positive proof that the dura mater or brain were injured. Of these 41 cases, 7 terminated fatally, one from abscess of liver, one from typhus, 2 from primary encephalitis through neglect of antiphlogistic treatment, 2 from phlebitis encephalica, one from secondary encephalitis, in consequence of the patient visiting a public house. Of the 34 cured, one only was trephined by Dr. Ross, and this, says Dr. S., was the only case of trephining which gave a favorable result in all three campaigns. Notwithstanding the operation—several days after the injury—seven venesections and sixty leeches were necessary to com bat the continuing inflammation of the brain, and Dr. S. attributes his recovery to this, and not to the operation. He has not, on principle, trephined in two campaigns. He advises that gunshot wounds of the head, should, in their recent state, be examined with great care, by the aid of the finger or the probe alone. They must not, at first, be dilated, under any pretext whatever, whether for the sake of diagnosis or of prophylactic treatment. He insists that great care should be taken not to let the right period for venesection pass by. He advises the *cautious* extraction of perfectly loose fragments and foreign bodies, but the removal of impacted balls should not be attempted.

Mr. Macleod states, that many surgeons of large experience, in the Crimea, allowed loose pieces of bone on the dura mater, to be thrown out by nature, and were not particular even about keeping the wound open. He believes this practice to be dangerous, and says that loose portions of bone should always be cautiously removed. He reports the following case as illustrating the evil effects of leaving them, as well as the injurious influence of too early a recurrence to a stimulant diet.

M'Louchlin, a private in the Connaught rangers, aged 19, was admitted into the general hospital on the 8th September. He had been knocked down, and rendered insensible, by a blow from a piece of shell in the final assault on the Redan. A scalp wound two and a half inches long, was found extending from before, backward over the vertex of the head, and a small piece of bone was observed to be depressed at its anterior extremity. The patient did not become conscious for twenty-four hours after admission. Purging, and low diet comprised his treatment. Cold dressing, and nothing else, was applied to the wound. He remained perfectly well, complaining only of slight headache and giddiness, for three months; small pieces of bone being discharged in the meantime from the wound, which had almost closed. After being about a month in hospital, he was allowed full diet, and a gill of grog daily. On the 8th of December, three months after receiving his wound, he complained of a sort of transient paralysis of the left arm, which, although it continued only for a second or two at a time, recurred frequently. His sense of smell, too, suddenly left him. There was no other symptom. On being questioned, he said he had had a rigor, and several "fainting fits" during the days immediately preceding that on which he first complained of the paralysis. Next day he said he had a more prolonged fit of paralysis during the night, than he ever had had before, the attack being preceded by pain in the left side. I first saw him during an attack on the 9th of December, which was more severe and more prolonged than any preceding one. His left arm hung powerless, and there was complete anæsthesia of the left arm and side, from the clavicle to the false ribs, and from the line of the nipple to the spine. The left side of the neck, behind the sterno-mastoid, was also without sensation. His face was unaffected. The integuments around the wound were puffy, and very sensitive. He said that his uneasy feelings had gradually increased as the wound closed. His bowels were opened freely, and a light poultice was applied to the wound, which was incised. The fit he had on the 9th passed off, leaving the arm weak. The sensibility of the left side slowly returned during the succeeding days. The fits of paralysis came and went, his arm recovering its power, in a great measure, between them. A sharp bit of bone was at last observed, lying on the dura mater, and when it was removed, the untoward symptoms disappeared. Shortly after this he came under my care. By quiet, and the use of unstimulating food and laxatives, he progressed most favorably; but on several occasions transient feelings of weakness—for there never again was a state of paralysis established—passed over the left side, when any scale of bone became loose, and lay on the dura mater, and, so soon as this was removed, these feelings left. If his bowels became costive, even for a very short time, not only did the headache and giddiness increase, but the numbness in the side returned. When he left for England no bits of bone could be discovered, and the wound was nearly closed; and he is now, I understand, doing duty with his regiment. Many of the symptoms, in this case, were those set down as calling for the use of the trephine; but the cautious removal of the fragments when loose, the local bleeding, and the purging, did all that was required.

As to the extraction of balls when lodged in the brain, Mr. Macleod remarks that the plain path of duty is to remove such foreign bodies, if practicable. Our boldness must not partake of temerity, he adds, yet all reasonable attempts ought to be made for their extraction. If the ball has penetrated deeply into the brain, he thinks it a matter of little moment what steps are taken; perhaps, however, it is the best line of conduct to let the man die in peace. He has never known a case of perforating gunshot wound of the head to recover, although such cases have been recorded. When signs of inflammatory or excited action supervene, he recommends instant and copious bleeding. He has never seen any good arise from the use of tartar emetic in these cases. Cold locally, purgatives, low diet, and early bleeding, repeated freely when signs of disturbance showed themselves, with the application, in some cases, of leeches to the head, seemed always sufficient, and, as he believes, are the most useful means of treating such patients. The trephine, saw, or elevator, should be had recourse to only in cases of fracture with great depression, where the bone is forced deeply into the brain, or when spiculæ, balls, or foreign bodies are impacted, and can not be removed through the wound by means of the forceps. The cases which call for operation secondarily, are those in which a foreign body is at this period discovered irritating the brain, and which can not be extracted without a piece of the bone being removed; or those in which signs of compression set in after a well-marked rigor, and continue to increase in intensity in spite of treatment, and have lasted for some time. The finger alone, and that cautiously, should be used in the examination, and if the bone is so extensively injured and depressed as to demand early interference, it will be sufficiently evident without incising the scalp for exploration. He does not agree with Stromeyer, who warns us particularly against attempting too soon to remove pieces of necrosed bone, as he thinks they do little harm, if allowed to remain. With this, Macleod's observation by no means coincides, and if the dead bone can be removed without violence, he thinks it should always be done as soon as it is found to be loose. He regards the after management of gunshot wounds of the head as most important; no class of cases, indeed, requiring more lengthened and careful supervision. Irregularities in diet, constipation, etc., may cause relapses long after the patient is apparently beyond danger. Many cases, he observes, are on record in which men with balls imbedded in the brain have apparently recovered completely, but have suddenly fallen down dead when they became intoxicated or excited.

CHAPTER IX.

WOUNDS OF ARTERIES.

Under this head, we shall consider those lesions of the arterial walls which are produced by external violence, and which may or may not give rise to a solution of continuity; in other words, which are penetrating or non-penetrating. The round form, the elastic coats, and the mobility of arteries, except where they pass directly over bone, enable them often to escape serious injury, even when a ball passes through an important region, like the neck or axilla. In the Crimean war, the neck was injured by gunshot more or less severely 128 times, and yet only 4 deaths resulted from these wounds. Contusion of a large artery may lead to such a diminution of its calibre, and the formation of coagula, as to cause its complete obliteration, and the mortification of the limb to which it is distributed. One of the most striking illustrations of the effect of a contusion of a large artery has been furnished us by Mr. Guthrie, and the preparation is still to be seen in the museum at Fort Pitt, Chatham, England. The specimen was taken from Private P. Tumbrill, of the grenadiers of the 74th regiment, who was wounded by a musket ball, passing from the inside to the outside of the middle of the thigh. The wound was inflicted on the 10th of April, 1814. On the 18th, the toes were affected with gangrene; on the 26th, it had extended above the ankle, and the patient died that night. The autopsy showed that the ball had passed between the artery and vein, at the point where the vein is situated partly behind it, and adheres only by the cellular membrane, through which the ball had made its passage. The coats of the vein were but little injured, while those of the artery were bruised. The artery here was much contracted in size, and filled above and below by coagula, rendering it impervious to the passage of blood.

Writers on civil surgery have united in referring to the great rarity of penetrating wounds of large arteries met with in private or in hospital practice, and have supposed that it was only on the battle field or in military hospitals that the surgeon could have a wide scope for observation; but the error of such an inference will be obvious after perusing Mr. Macleod's History of the Crimean War, in which he states that military surgeons are seldom required to treat wounds of large arteries, only 15 cases having presented for treatment among the 4,434 wounded in that war. This statement may, at first view, be regarded as in direct contradiction to the remark of Sir Geo. Ballingall, that "three fourths of those killed in battle are supposed to die from the escape or extravasation of blood." The appparent discrepancy has been well explained by Macleod himself. He admits that it is unquestionable that a large number of the dead sink from hemorrhage. A great artery is shot through, and in a moment the heart has emptied itself of blood, the very nature of the wounds, in most of these cases, causing death very rapidly, and giving the surgeon but little opportunity for treatment.

Contusion merely may lead to such a diminution in the calibre of an artery and the formation of coagula as in the end to cause its obliteration, and gangrene of the limb nourished by it. An artery of the size of the brachial or femoral, when divided to the extent of one third or one fourth of its circumference, does not heal without rendering it impervious. An artery like the radial or temporal, when completely divided is less likely to bleed than when it is only half divided, as it can neither retract nor contract. Military writers differ as to the frequency of primary hemorrhage on the battle-field. The frequency is affected by the speed of the ball; if diminished, the contusion is more likely to favor secondary hemorrhage; if in full flight, it may so divide the artery as to give rise to immediate and speedily fatal bleeding. An artery opened by a gunshot wound may bleed profusely for a few moments, and then be arrested by faintness, after which it may not reappear for days or weeks. The longest period mentioned is seven weeks. Of course, no patient can be pronounced safe until the wound has healed. Whatever may be thought, in civil practice, of styptics, or compression, as a means of arresting hemorrhage from arteries of a medium size, the military surgeon will often be so situated that he can trust to the ligature alone. Should the hemorrhage have ceased at the time of his arrival, although disposed to bow to the high authority of Mr. Guthrie in other matters, he may still feel unwilling to subject the patient to the fearful risk he may incur from a second hemorrhage, especially if the artery wounded be large, and he will, therefore, proceed to secure the bleeding vessel. With a large number of wounded requiring his care, the surgeon may be unable, on the recurrence of hemorrhage, to render necessary aid, and the patient might perish from adhering too literally to the rule, never to ligate a wounded artery unless it is bleeding at the time of the operation. Mr. Macleod is thus emphatic upon this point: "Not to interfere unless the vessel is bleeding, must not always be understood too literally, or we will often be prevented from performing the operation till our patient is beyond our help. The hemorrhage recurs over and over again, and the surgeon, though as near as is practicable, arrives only in time to see the bed drenched, and the patient and attendant intensely alarmed. There is, at the moment, no bleeding, and he vainly hopes there will be no return; and so, on goes the game between ebbing life and menacing death, the loss not great at each time, but mighty in the sum, till all assistance is useless. Many a valuable life has thus been lost, which might have been saved by a more decided course of action."

Admit that in some cases when the bleeding has ceased, it has never returned, and that in others after the operation, the collateral circulation has never been re-established, and gangrene of the extremity the result, yet we know that even Mr. Guthrie's own objection to the ligature of a wounded artery, on the cardiac side of the opening alone, is based upon the well ascertained fact, that the collateral circulation is too often sufficient to maintain the hemorrhage from the distal side, and thus destroy the patient. If such are the almost certain consequences to be dreaded, after the operation on the cardiac side, surely the patient, in many cases, incurs less risk of death from mortification, the result of a deficient supply of blood, than for a repetition of the hemorrhage which (though not bleeding at the time), with the very next gush of blood may prove immediately fatal.

But we object only to the too rigid enforcement of Mr. Guthrie's rule. If the patient can be watched by competent assistants, for days and weeks, until the wound has healed, then, of course, there can be no impropriety in deferring the operation until the wounded artery bleeds through the external wound, or the blood becomes infiltrated into the surrounding tissues.

An artery may be but partially penetrated by a wound, and the reliance to be placed upon the healing of such an injury may be inferred from the following case reported by Mr. Guthrie, in his Treatise on Wounds and Injuries of Arteries. A gentleman cut his throat with a razor, and fell bathed in blood. The bleeding was arrested by thrusting sponges into the wound. The left carotid was laid bare, and the internal jugular was wounded, giving rise to the principal bleeding. A tenaculum was passed through the edges of the opening in the vein. and they were drawn together by a single silk thread, so as to close the opening. The ends of the ligature were cut off close to the knot. The carotid was clearly seen by the side of the vein, having a transverse mark or cut upon it, which did not appear to penetrate beyond the middle coat; and after due consideration, it was presumed that this wound might heal, without requiring a ligature to be placed upon the artery. On the eighth day arterial hemorrhage took place, and Mr. Guthrie at once tied the carotid below the opening, but in consequence of the reflux from the head, the flow of blood was but little diminished by the operation. On attempting to apply another ligature above the opening, Mr. G. found what he had suspected, that the wound was immediately below the division of the common carotid, into the external and internal carotid arteries. The hemorrhage ceased on placing a ligature on the external carotid, above the wound, and as the patient was greatly exhausted, the internal carotid was not tied. The bleeding did not return, but the patient died next morning from exhaustion. The lesson taught by the above case, says Mr. G., is, that where an opening is made into a vein, of the size of the internal jugular (its division not being complete), a ligature may be made to include the cut portion without interfering with the canal of the vessel; and that when the two outer coats of a large artery are divided, it will be better to place a ligature above and below the injured part at once, rather than leave it to the efforts of nature.

A mere puncture of an artery as by the point of a tenaculum, has given rise to such hemorrhage as to require the ligature. Mr. Guthrie saw several such cases in which ulceration caused secondary hemorrhage, demanding an operation. A large puncture, or a longitudinal slit, of from one to two lines in extent, says Mr. G. does not commonly unite, except under pressure, although the edges of the wound may separate, so as to allow blood to issue in any quantity. It sometimes oozes out, and occasionally does not do even that, unless some obstacle to the circulation takes place, when the blood is propelled with a jet, and the edges of the cut having been once separated, blood continues to be thrown forth in considerable quantity. Mr. Guthrie himself is compelled to admit that *no* reliance can be placed on the efforts of nature, in healing a wound in an artery in man, and yet because it does "occasionally occur" (to use his own language), he lays down the rule that "no operation is to be performed on any artery, unless it bleeds at the moment of its performance, inasmuch as hemorrhage once suppressed may never return!"

When there is a long rent in an artery, or when it is divided through half of its circumference, its retractile and contractile powers only enlarge the wound, and interfere or entirely prevent the closing of the opening. Again, a foreign body remaining in the wound will have the same effect. The effect of extracting a ball, in some of the latter cases, is well shown in the following case, where the vertebral was tied by M. M. Maisonneuve and Favrot, February 20, 1852. The operation was performed for the purpose of arresting a serious hemorrhage produced by a gunshot wound in the cervical region. The method adopted, we copy from the Union Medicale, March 20, 1852. An incision of about fifteen centimetres was made along the anterior border of the sterno-mastoid muscle, a little external to the opening made by the entrance of the ball. This exposed the carotid artery and the internal jugular vein intact. It was easy, through this opening, to discover, First, the cricoid cartilage, the left side of which had been grazed. Second, the upper rings of the trachea, and the œsophagus which had been exposed, but not injured by the ball. In exploring the bottom of the wound for the vessel which furnished the hemorrhage, the ball was discovered in the body of the sixth cervical vertebra, and was immediately extracted. The hemorrhage at once became violent, and appeared to proceed from the vertebral artery, which had been wounded in the canal of the transverse processes of the vertebræ. At length the wounded vessel was discovered, and was seized with a spring forceps. The facility with which this was done, led them to suppose that they had been deceived, and that instead of having secured the vertebral artery, they had found only some branch of the inferior thyroid. An armed needle, with a very short curve, was passed around the vessel, which was tied above and below the wound. The hemorrhage was immediately and completely arrested.

Another vessel, more superficial, which was proved to be the inferior thyroid, was afterward tied without difficulty, as were several others of minor importance. Matters progressed favorably, and on the 29th of February, the ligatures came away. On the 5th of March, fever suddenly manifested itself with violent mental disturbance. On the 9th of March, at 2 o'clock P. M. while making his toilet, the patient was seized with a severe pain in the cervical region, uttered a cry, and instantly fell in a profound coma, which lasted until 9 o'clock in the evening, when he died. At the autopsy, the vertebral artery, for an inch above and below the wound, was filled with a solid coagulum.

The body of the vertebra was hollowed by a deep canal, the extremity of which communicated with the spinal canal, by a small opening evidently produced in the last moments of life. The spongy tissue of the bone was infiltrated with pus, and a sero-purulent exudation existed in the spinal canal, both in the external cellular tissue and in the sub-serous tissue of the envelopes of the spinal marrow. No other serious lesion was discovered in any of the other organs.

In connection with the above, the following are also worthy of record:

A fragment of tobacco-pipe, entering by the mouth, pierced the anterior pillar of the fauces on the right side, and lodged. Hemorrhage took place at the time, but stopped of itself; and I saw the young man six or seven hours afterward, pale, and with one tonsil swollen near the wound. I could not see or feel the fragment of pipe, nor could I detect it in the wound with a probe. A large swelling formed in the upper half of the neck, which, on the seventh day suddenly began to pulsate, while arterial blood issued copiously from the mouth. The carotid was tied below the swelling. The operation was immediately followed by paralysis of the left extremities, and it persisted. On the thirteenth day after the accident, bleeding suddenly recurred through the mouth, and was immediately fatal. At the post-mortem examination, the lower end of the fragment of pipe was found lying in a hole at the top of the common carotid, surrounded with buff-colored lymph, and with a carotid branch on each side of it. The wound of the vessel could not possibly have closed. Although the primitive carotid was filled with clot from near the wound down to the ligature, the external and internal carotids were empty. There were also several fœtid abscesses in the right hemisphere of the cerebrum. In reporting this case, Mr. Vincent remarks, that if the piece of pipe had been discovered and extracted through the mouth, fatal hemorrhage would, in all probability, have followed, as he believed to have occurred in a previous and similar case. The most embarrassing cases to which a surgeon can be called, are those where a wound has been inflicted in the vicinity of the division of a large artery, as, for example, the bifurcation of the carotid-brachial near the elbow joint, and the popliteal as it divides into the posterior and anterior tibial. Great perplexity must often exist as to the source of the hemorrhage, and of the propriety of attempting to apply a ligature above and below the wound.

We might mention a number of instances in which the most skillful and experienced surgeons have ligated a main arterial trunk, for a wound of a comparatively unimportant branch. Roux, in his Quarante Annees de Pratique Chirurgicale, relates the details of a case in which both Boyer and himself, made a mistake, and applied a ligature to the femoral, to arrest hemorrhage, which was afterward proved by a post mortem, to be due to a wound of the superior articular branch of the popliteal, and the patient perished from mortification. He reports another case where at first he supposed the popliteal had been wounded, but although the hemorrhage was arrested by *tamponnement*, purulent arthritis supervened, and destroyed the patient.

On examination, the opening was found in the superior articular branch. The famous case of Captain Seton who was wounded in a duel, and treated by Mr. Liston, is still fresh in the memory of every surgeon. Mr. Liston committed the, perhaps, fatal error of applying a ligature to the external iliac, to cure a supposed false aneurism, which proved to be a collection of blood from a branch, distributed to the abdominal walls. Mr. Guthrie gives the following case, treated by Staff Surgeon Collier:—H. B., 44th regiment, aged 20, was wounded by a spear or sword, on the 17th of June, which passed in at the angle of the left jaw, and penetrated the mouth, lacerating the tongue severely in three or four places. He was brought into the hospital in Brussels, on the 19th, and had, by his account, lost a considerable quantity of blood on the way. On the evening of the 22d, I found arterial blood jetting up with considerable force from the bottom of a narrow deep wound, and flowing in different directions, as if from several branches of the external carotid. I attempted dilatation; but, as all efforts to trace the sources of bleeding were fruitless, I applied, steadily and forcibly, graduated compresses, moderating the flow of blood, by compresses on the carotid. Although the hemorrhage yielded for three or four minutes, it was soon evident that it had changed its channel for it, began to flow as furiously through the mouth as it before had done through the wound, and the coagula required to be constantly removed to prevent suffocation. My opinion being, that the patient's preservation depended on securing the common carotid artery; I performed the operation at 8 o'clock that evening; the hemorrhage ceased the instant the ligature was applied. In two hours after the operation, the patient was quite tranquil and sensible: the pulse feeble; countenance very pale. On the following morning (23d), I found him perfectly sensible and easy, with the exception of some sense of heat in the throat, rather increased since the operation; the pulse was 96, with slight sharpness: no appearance of hemorrhage. On the 5th of July, the ligature came away, and on the 12th of August, he was discharged cured, having suffered only from two slight attacks of erysipelas of the face, which gave no uneasiness. Roux informs us that he once applied a ligature to the common carotid for a gunshot wound of the mouth, by which the right lingual artery was divided; and we might give many other cases of a similar nature, but time and space forbid.

With the exception of Dr. Thomson, in his Report of Observations made in the Military Hospitals, in Belgium, we know of no writer who has devoted, to the subject of consecutive hemorrhage, so much attention. The destruction of the vitality of the arterial coats by gunshot wounds, would lead us to suspect much trouble from secondary hemorrhage, the result of sloughing, but Roux's observations of the wounded during the three memorable days in July 1830, taught him that this hemorrhage, after an interval of some days or weeks, is not always due to the sloughing process, but to the ulceration following the irritation of bony spiculæ or fragments. Sometimes, again, it may be due to the enlarged capillaries. When it is due to the separation of an eschar, which, according to his experience, generally occurs from the eighth to the tenth day. This consecutive hemorrhage may appear without any warning, at other times there may be a serous discharge of a reddish tinge, a discoloration of the integuments, and a condition of the parts but little favorable to the operation of ligating both ends of the wounded vessel.

Mr. Macleod remarks, that in the Crimea, these cases were the cause of extreme anxiety, as the deteriorated state of the health of their patients made such an accident peculiarly disastrous. Their strength could not withstand such a drain. Where an opportunity was afforded for treatment, tonics, as quinine and iron, were of the most service.

Although the general precepts with which Mr. Guthrie concludes his work On Wounds and Injuries of the Arteries, may, in some particulars, be open to dispute, yet the cordial indorsement they now receive from the profession, is sufficient evidence of their great practical value, and we know we confer a great favor upon those who can not have access to his treatise by their republication.

GUTHRIE'S GENERAL CONCLUSIONS.

1. The Hunterian operation for the cure of an aneurism is not applicable to the treatment of a wounded artery, inasmuch as the wound of the artery communicates with the external parts, and nothing intervenes to prevent blood flowing from the wound in its side, or from its cut extremities.

2. When a large artery is divided and bleeds, the wound should be enlarged, if necessary, and a ligature placed on both the divided ends, but if the artery be only injured, and not quite divided, the ligatures should be applied, one immediately above, the other below the injured part. The artery may or may not be then cut across, at the pleasure of the operator, but the limb or part should be placed in a relaxed position. A bandage should not be applied, and the edges of the wound should be simply brought together by adhesive plasters, which do not extend completely round the limb.

3. No operation is to be performed on any artery unless it bleeds at the moment of the performance, inasmuch as hemorrhage, once suppressed, may never return.

4. The intervention of muscular fibers, or of whole muscles, is not a sufficient reason for tying the artery at a distant part. They must be divided, if it be possible, to the extent required for a due exposure of the injured artery, and its accompanying veins and nerves.

5. If the wound pass indirectly to the principal artery, from the back of the thigh, for instance, to the femoral artery in front, or from the outside of the arm to the humeral artery on the inside, the surgeon may (on satisfying himself of the part likely to be injured by the introduction of a probe), cut down on the vessel opposite the part supposed to be wounded, by the most simple and approved method. When the artery is exposed, the probe will point out the spot at which the vessel has, in all probability, been wounded. Pressure made below this spot on the artery, will cause it to be distended and to bleed, if the flow of blood be not prevented from above. The artery is then to be secured by two ligatures, and the lower one should, if possible, be applied first.

6. The tourniquet should never be used in an operation for aneurism, or for a wounded artery. Compression by the hand, in the course of a wounded vessel, is allowable.

7. The blood from the upper end of a divided artery, or that nearest the heart, is of a scarlet arterial color.

8. The blood from the lower end of a divided artery, or that which is farthest from the heart, is of a dark or venous color, when it happens to flow immediately after the division of the vessel. At a subsequent period, it may assume more of the color of arterial blood, but it rarely does so for several days after the receipt of the injury, and always flows, or at least until a very late period, in a continuous stream.

9. This regurgitation or flow of blood from the lower end of a divided artery is a favorable sign, inasmuch as it shows that the collateral circulation will probably be sufficient to maintain the life of the extremity.

10. The collateral circulation is in almost every instance capable of maintaining the life of the upper extremity when the axillary artery is divided, and the color of the blood which flows from the end of the artery, on its being divided, is not always as dark as in the lower extremity, and it sooner resumes its arterial color.

11. The collateral circulation is not always capable of maintaining the life of the limb when the femoral artery is injured. The best assistance which art can give is to rub the foot and leg in the gentlest manner, between the hands of one or two strong young women, for several hours, or even for the first three or four days; relaxing this process very little even during sleep. When the vein is divided at the same time, or rendered impervious, the limb usually mortifies.

12. The collateral circulation is sufficient to maintain the life of an extremity in almost every case in which an aneurism has existed for eight or ten weeks, although it may be incapable of doing this if the principal artery has been suddenly divided, without any previous disease having existed in the part.

13. The theory and the operation for aneurism are never to be applied to the treatment of a wounded artery, which has caused a diffused or circumscribed aneurism, *while the external wound communicates with the artery*, unless it be impossible or impracticable to tie the bleeding vessel.

14. When an artery has been wounded, and the external opening has healed for weeks or months, so as to give rise to a diffused or circumscribed aneurism, it may be treated according to the theory of aneurism occurring from an internal cause, if the case will permit it without danger; although with this difference, that as the artery is sound the operation may be performed close to the tumor. If any doubt exist as to the capability of the collateral circulation to

support the life of the lower extremity, after the external iliac has been secured by ligature, the operation should be performed at the injured part by opening the swelling and enlarging the wound, as in the case of a wounded artery.

15. When a circumscribed or diffused aneurism which has formed after a wound has been opened, whether by accident or design, it is placed in the situation of a wounded artery, and should be treated as such. If the aneurism has arisen from disease of the vessel, and the wound or opening into it cannot be permanently closed, the limb is in a worse state than if the artery had been wounded by accident; because a ligature or ligatures placed on a diseased artery are little likely to be successful. They are liable to all the difficulties and inconveniences attendant on the old operation of aneurism. If a case of the kind should occur in a popliteal or femoral aneurism, situated at or below where the artery passes between the triceps and the bone, amputation, if it can be done low down, will be the best remedy. If the aneurism should have formed higher up, and the opening can be closed with any prospect of its healing; a ligature may be placed upon the artery above it; but on the recurrence of hemorrhage which can not be restrained by moderate pressure, the artery must be tied below, or recourse had to amputation. It is, however, to be observed, that amputation under these circumstances, when resorted to as a third operation, rarely succeeds.

16. When an artery is wounded with a simple fracture of a bone, or with a comminuted fracture of smaller bones, with an external communicating opening, both ends of the artery should be secured, and the limb treated in the usual manner.

17. When the bone broken is the femur, and the artery divided is the femoral artery, the operation of amputation will generally be advisable. It will always be so, if the fracture is a comminuted one, or the shaft of the bone is extensively splintered.

18. When the broken bone injures the artery, and gives rise to an aneurism, the treatment is to be, first of the fracture and then of the aneurism, as soon as circumstances render it advisable or necessary to have recourse to the operation for aneurism; which can only be after time has been given for the collateral branches to enlarge, so as to maintain the life of the limb.

19. When mortification takes place in addition to, or as a consequence of, a wounded artery, amputation should be had recourse to forthwith.

20. The place of operation should be, in almost all cases, at the seat of the original wound; but there may be an exception, viz:

21. When, for instance, the injury has been a mere cut, just sufficient to divide the artery and vein immediately below Poupart's ligament, and mortification of the foot supervenes, amputation should then be performed below the knee, or at the part where mortification more usually stops for a time.

This rule is founded on the observation, that great efforts are made by nature to arrest mortification a little below the knee. Sometimes they succeed; when they fail, death is almost inevitable. The advice to amputate at this part is founded on the fact of its being infinitely less dangerous when done there than on the thigh, independently of saving a joint.

22. When mortification has *continued for several days*, and is spreading, without having once stopped, the constitution of the patient being implicated as marked by fever, amputation should not be performed until the mortification has been arrested, and the line of separation has been well formed. In many cases, where there is great weakness or irritability of constitution, it will be advisable to defer the operation to a later period, particularly if there be hope of the patient's becoming stronger and more tranquil.

23. If the mortification has once stopped, and then begins again to spread, it will never again cease to extend, and amputation may give some chance of life.

24. Amputation of the arm should never be had recourse to in consequence of a wound of the axillary artery, unless mortification takes place.

25. When mortification takes place after the operation for aneurism, the surgeon must be guided by the state of the patient's constitution in resorting to or refraining from amputation.

26. When hemorrhage occurs from the surface of a stump, the artery should be tied at the part from which the blood comes in the first instance, if it can be easily done. If this should not suffice, the artery must be tied higher up, just at such distance as will afford a fair hope of its not having been affected by the derangement of the stump, which has led to the failure of consolidation in the extremity of the artery; yet not too high to admit of the junction of any large collateral branches. If the bleeding proceeds from several small vessels, and can not be arrested, the principal trunk should be tied immediately above the diseased part, and the patient removed to a

purer atmosphere, without which an operation rarely succeeds in any case.

27. When an aneurismal tumor mortifies, it is unnecessary and improper to tie the artery above the tumor, because it will be obliterated if the mortification be arrested by the efforts of nature, which the operation may interfere with, and even prevent, while, if the mortification spreads, it will be a matter of supererogation, and only hasten the patient's dissolution. When an aneurism inflames, is opened by ulceration, and bleeds profusely, so as not to be arrested, it is a proper case for amputation, if such an operation can be performed.

CHAPTER X.

ON THE USE OF CHLOROFORM.

(From Macleod's "Notes on the Surgery of the War in the Crimea.")

The advantages derived from the use of anæsthetics are perhaps more evident and more appreciated in the field than in civil practice. The many dreadful injuries which are presented to us in war, and the severe suffering which so often results from them, soon cause us fully to appreciate the benefits bestowed by such "pain-soothers."

The vast majority of the surgeons of the eastern army were most enthusiastic in their anticipations of what chloroform was to accomplish. It was expected to revolutionize the whole art of surgery. Many operations, hitherto discarded, were now to be performed; and many, which the experience of the Peninsula said were necessary, were henceforth to be done away with.

In the British army, chloroform was almost universally employed but although the French also used it very extensively, as we learn from Baudens, still I do not think, from what I saw of its employment in their hospitals, that they had our confidence in it. Baudens tells us* that "they had no fatal accident to deplore from its use, although during the eastern campaign chloroform was employed thirty thousand times, or more. In the Crimea alone," he continues, "it was administered to more than twenty thousand wounded, according to the calculations of M. Scrive."

In one division of our army it was not so commonly used as in the others, from an aversion to it entertained by the principal medical officer of the division—a gentleman of very extensive experience. The only case in which, with any show of fairness, fatal consequences could be said to have followed its use, occurred in the division referred to. The patient, a man thirty-two years of age, belonged to the 62d regiment, and was about to have a finger removed. The chloroform was administered on a handkerchief, as he sat in a chair. Death was sudden; and artificial respiration, which

* Revue des Deux Mondes, Apr. 1857.

was the means of resuscitation employed, failed to restore him. No pathological condition sufficient to account for death was found post-mortem. Some five or six other cases were brought forward by the small body of surgeons who were suspicious of the action of chloroform, as having ended fatally from its effects; but in none of these could, I think, the least pretext be found for the imputation, further than that the anæsthetic had been administered at some period previous to death. A man who had been dreadfully mutilated, and who had lost much blood, died shortly after having his thigh removed high up. Chloroform had been used, and to it was ascribed the fatal issue. Death, twenty or thirty hours after a capital operation, rendered necessary by the most dreadful injuries, must be attributed to the chloroform, and so on, and no note taken of the effects of severe injury, *plus* a capital operation, in shattering the already enfeebled powers! Death occurring under such circumstances, when no chloroform was employed, would not be thought to demand any special explanation, nor does the fact that the injury was occasioned by a round shot introduce any new element into the calculation.

The objections made to the use of chloroform were restricted to two classes of cases—trivial accidents, in which it was thought necessary to run the risk of giving it, and amputations of the thigh, in which a fatal accession of shock was feared. However this may be, it certainly shows the little practical force of these objections, that, while with every indulgence in the interpretation of the law "post hoc," etc., only some half dozen cases could be obtained throughout the whole army to illustrate the pernicious effects of this agent, and that, too, when thousands upon thousands had been submitted to its action, and hundreds of surgeons of equal experience to the objectors were ready to record their unqualified opinion in its favor, as well as their gratitude for its benefits. For my own part, I never had reason, for one moment, to doubt the unfailing good and universal applicability of chloroform in gunshot injuries, *if properly administered.* I most conscientiously believe that its use in our army directly saved very many lives—that many operations necessary for this end were performed by its assistance, which could not otherwise have been attempted—that these operations were more successfully, because more carefully, executed—that life was often saved even by the avoidance of pain—the *morale* of the wounded better sustained, and the courage and comfort of the surgeon increased. I think I have seen enough of its effects to conclude, that, if its action is not carried beyond the stage necessary for operation, it does not increase the depression which results from injury, but that, on the contrary, it in many instances supports the strength under operation. Its usefulness is seen in nothing more than when, by its employment, we perform operations close upon the receipt of injury, and thereby, if not entirely, at least in a great degree, are able to ward off that "embranlement" of the nervous system which is otherwise sure to follow, and whose nature we know only by its dire effects.

To men who had lost much blood, it had, of course, to be administered with great care, from the rapidity of its absorption in such persons; but if we do not act on broader principles in its exhibition than reckoning the number of drops which have been employed, or the part of the nervous system which we may presume to be at the time engaged, then we must expect disastrous results. It is difficult to see how its use could favor secondary hemorrhage after operation, as some said it did; but it is, on the contrary, easy to understand how the opposite result might follow. That purulent absorption should prevail among men so broken in health as our men were, need not be explained by the employment of chloroform; and that ice would prove more useful in the slighter operative cases in field practice, few will be disposed to admit, either on the ground of time, efficiency or opportunity. To Deputy Inspector-General Taylor we owe the practical observation, that chloroform appears to act more efficiently when administered in the open air.

In the prolonged searches which are sometimes necessary for the extraction of foreign bodies, chloroform is useful, not only preventing pain, but also in restraining muscular contractions, by which obstacles are thrown in the way of our extraction, which did not oppose themselves to the introduction of the body. Then much is gained in field practice by the mere avoidance of the patient's screams when undergoing operation, as it frequently happens that but a thin partition, a blanket or a few planks, intervene between him who is being operated upon, and those who wait to undergo a like trial. Thus, when, as after a general engagement, a vast number of men come in quick succession to be subjected to operation, it is a point of great importance to save them from the depression and dread which the screams and groans of their comrades necessarily produce in them.

It is, therefore, my clear conviction, that the experience of the late war, as regards chloroform, is uneqivocally favorable; that it has shown that chloroform, both directly and indirectly, saves life; that it abates a vast amount of suffering; that its use is as plainly indicated in gunshot as in other wounds; and that, if administered with equal care, it matters not whether the operation about to be performed be necessitated by a gunshot wound, or by any of the accidents which occur in civil life.

APPENDIX:

CONTAINING

SUPPLY TABLES; FORMS OF REQUISITIONS FOR SUPPLIES; RETURNS, ETC.

APPENDIX.

SUPPLY FOR MEDICAL OFFICER.

Each Medical Officer will be supplied with the following surgical instruments for his personal use, which he will retain in his immediate possession so long as he remains in the Army, and for the complete and serviceable condition of which at all times he will be held responsible :

AMPUTATING.

1 Capital Saw.
1 Metacarpal Saw.
1 Capital Amputating Knife.
1 Medium " "
1 Small " "
1 Large Catling.
1 Small "
1 Scalpel.
1 Tenaculum.
1 Artery Needle.
1 " Forceps.
1 Bone "
1 Spiral Tourniquet.
12 Surgeon's Needles.
1 Mahogany Case, brass bound.
1 Gutta Percha Pouch.

TREPHINING.

2 Trephines.
1 Scalpel, with Raspitor.
1 Heys' Saw.
1 Elevator.
1 Brush.
I Mahogany Case, brass bound.

EXSECTING.

1 Bone Forceps, Liston's.
2 Bone Forceps, sharp, assorted.
1 Bone Forceps, for sequestra.
1 Chain Saw.
1 Chisel.
1 Gouge.
1 Lenticular Knife.
2 Spatulas, protecting.
1 Trephine, small crown.
1 Ecraseur.
1 Mahogany Case, brass bound.
1 Gutta Perch Pouch.

GENERAL OPERATING.

1 Metacarpal Saw.
1 Trocar.
1 Ball Forceps.
1 Gullet "
1 Artery "
1 Dressing Forceps.
2 Scissors, straight, and curved.
1 Artery Needle, with 4 points.
12 Surgeon's Needles.
1 Tourniquet.
1 Small Amputating Knife.
1 " Catling.
3 Bistouries.
1 Hernia Knife.
3 Scalpels.
1 Cataract Knife.
1 " Needle.
1 Tenaculum.
1 Double Hook.
6 Steel Bougies, silv'd, double curve, Nos. 1 and 2, 3 and 4, 5 and 6, 7 and 8, 9 and 10, 11 and 12.
6 Wax Bougies, Nos. 2, 4, 6, 8, 10.
3 Silver Catheters, Nos. 3, 6, 9.
6 Gum-elastic Catheters, Nos. 1, 3, 5, 7, 9, 11.
2 Mahogany Cases, brass bound.
1 Gutta Percha Pouch.

POCKET.

1 Large Scalpel.
1 Small "
1 Artery Forceps.

1 Bull-dog "
1 Curved "
1 Dressing "
1 Needle.
1 Sharp-pointed Bistoury.
1 Probe-pointed "
1 Long Probe-pointed Bistoury.
1 Straight Scissors.
1 Knee "
1 Flat-curved Scissors.
1 Gum lancet.
1 Tenaculum.
1 Tenotomy Knife.
1 Abscess Lancet.
1 Exploring Needle.
1 Exploring Trocar.
1 Seton Needle.
1 Spatula.
2 Probes.
1 Director.
1 Double Canula.
1 Comp'd Silver Catheter.
6 Surgeon's Needles
1 Artery Needle.
1 Morocco Case.
1 Leather Trunk.

To each General and Post Hospital, one ounce of *brominium*, with printed directions for preparing and administering Bibron's antidote to the poison of *serpents*. Also one bottle of *liquor ferri per sulphatis*, and one bottle of *liquor ammoniæ*, in equal proportions, with printed directions for preparing speedily and for administering the *hydrated sesqui-oxide of iron*, as an antidote to poisoning by *arsenic*.

If the following articles of Hospital Furniture can not be obtained with the hospital fund, they may be procured from a quartermaster, or medical disbursing officer, by special requisition :

ARTICLES.

Basins, wash.
Bowls.
Brushes.
Buckets.
Candlesticks.
Clothes-lines.
Cups.
Dippers and Ladles.
Graters.
Gridirons.
Kettles, tea.
Knives and Forks.
Lamps and Lanterns.
Locks and Keys.
Mugs.
Pans, frying.
" sauce.
Pitchers.
Plates and Dishes.
Pots, chamber and chair.
" coffee and tea.
Sadirons.
Shovels, fire
Snuffers.
Spoons.
Tongs and Pokers.
Tumblers.
Woodsaws.

STANDARD SUPPLY TABLE FOR FIELD SERVICE.

ARTICLES.		QUANTITIES.			MEMORANDA.
		Reg't 3 mos.	Bat. 3 mos.	Com. 3 mos.	
MEDICINES.					
Acidi acetici,	lb.	1	½	½	
" sulph. aromatici,	lb.	1	½	¼	
" tannici,	oz.	2	1	1	
Alcoholis,	cong.	2	1	½	
Aluminis,	lb.	1	½	¼	
Ammoniæ carbonatis,	oz.	16	8	4	
Antimonii et potass. tartratis,	oz.	2	1	1	
Argenti nitratis (crystals),	oz.	2	1	½	
" " (fused),	oz.	2	1	½	
Brominii,	oz.	1	1	1	
Camphoræ,	lb.	4	2	1	
Ceræ albæ,	oz.	2	2	1	
Cerati resinæ,	lb.	2	1	½	
" simplicis,	lb.	8	4	2	
Chloroformi,	lb.	2	1	1	
Copaibæ,	lb.	2	1	½	
Creasoti,	oz.	2	1	1	
Cupri sulphatis,	oz.	4	2	1	
Emplastri adhæsivi,	yds.	10	5	3	

Emplastri cantharidis,	lb.	4	2	1
" ichthyocollæ,	yds.	10	5	3
Extracti belladonnæ,	oz.	1	1	1
" buchu fluidi,	lb.	1	½	¼
" colchici acetici,	oz.	2	1	1
" colocynthidis comp.,	oz.	16	8	4
" glycyrrhizæ,	lb.	2	1	½
" rhei fluidi,	lb.	2	1	½
" senegæ fluidi,	oz.	8	4	4
" sennæ fluidi,	lb.	2	1	½
Ferri per sulphatis,	oz.	4	2	1
Hydrargyri chloridi corrosivi,	oz.	½	½	½
" " mitis,	lb.	2	1	½
Iodinii,	oz.	4	2	1
Liquoris ammoniæ,	lb.	4	2	1
" potass. arsenitis,	oz.	4	2	1
Magnesiæ sulphatis,	lb.	20	10	5
Massæ pil: hydragyri,	oz.	16	8	4
Morphiæ sulphatis,	dr.	4	2	1
Olei caryophylii,	oz.	1	1	1
" menthæ piperitæ,	oz.	2	1	1
" olivæ,	bott.	8	4	2
" ricini,	qt. bott.	12	6	3
" terebinthinæ,	qt. bott.	8	4	2
" tiglii,	dr.	2	1	1
Pilul: cathartic: comp.: (U. S.),	doz.	8	4	2
" opii (U. S.),	doz.	8	4	2
" quiniæ sulphatis (3 grs.),	doz.	8	4	2
Plumbi acetatis,	lb.	2	1	½
Potassæ bicarbonatis,	lb.	1	½	¼
" chloratis,	lb.	2	1	½
" nitratis,	lb.	1	½	¼
Potassii cyanureti,	dr.	1	1	1
" iodidi,	oz.	8	4	2

TABLE FOR FIELD SERVICE—*Continued.*

ARTICLES.		QUANTITIES. Reg't 3 mos.	Bat. 3 mos.	Com. 3 mos.	MEMORANDA.
MEDICINES—*Continued.*					
Pulveris acaciæ,	lb.	4	2	1	
" capsici,	lb.	½	¼	¼	
" ipecacuanhæ,	lb.	1	½	¼	
" " et opii,	oz.	8	4	4	
" lini,	lb.	16	8	4	
" opii,	lb.	2	1	½	
" rhei,	lb.	½	¼	¼	
" sinapis nigræ,	lb.	12	6	3	
Quiniæ sulphatis,	oz.	24	12	6	
Sacchari,	lb.	10	5	2	
Saponis,	lb.	8	4	2	
Sodæ bicarbonatis,	lb.	1	½	¼	
Spiritus ammoniæ aromatici,	oz.	4	2	2	
" ætheris comp.	lb.	1	½	½	
" " nitrici,	lb.	2	1	½	
" vini gallici,	bott.	24	12	6	
Strychniæ,	dr.	1	1	1	
Tincturæ, aconiti radicis,	lb.	1	½	¼	
" ferri chloridi,	lb.	1	½	¼	

Tincturæ opii,	oz.	16	8	6	
" veratri viridis,	oz.	8	4	2	
Unguenti hydrargyri,	lb.	1	½	¼	
" " nitratis,	lb.	½	¼	¼	
Zinci acetatis,	oz.	2	1	1	
Zinci sulphatis,	oz.	2	1	1	
INSTRUMENTS.					
Buck's instrument for the throat,	no.	1	1	1	
Cupping glasses and tins,	no.	16	8	4	Half glass, half tin.
Lancets, spring,	no.	1	1	1	
" thumb (with cases),	no.	6	4	2	
Pocket,	sets.	1	1	1	
Probangs, whalebone,	no.	12	6	2	
Scarificators,	no.	4	2	1	
Splints (major),	sets.	1	1	1	
Stomach pump and case,	no.	1	1	1	
Syringes, enema,	no.	4	2	1	
" penis, glass,	no.	8	4	2	l Davidson's; 1 hard rubber, 6 oz.
" " India-rubber,	no.	8	4	2	
Teeth extracting,	sets.	1	1	1	
Tongue depressor (hinge),	no.	1	1	1	
Tourniquets, field,	no.	8	4	2	
" spiral,	no.	2	2	1	
Trusses, hernia,	no.	6	3	2	
BOOKS.					
Anatomy (surgical),	cop.	1	1	1	
Medical Practice,	cop.	1	1	1	
Regulations for Medical Department,	cop.	1	1	1	
Surgery (operative),	cop.	1	1	1	
Thompson's Conspectus,	cop.	2	1	1	

TABLE FOR FIELD SERVICE—*Continued.*

ARTICLES.		QUANTITIES. Reg't 3 mos.	Bat. 3 mos.	Com. 3 mos.	MEMORANDA.
BOOKS—*Continued.*					
Blank,	no.	4	4	4	
HOSPITAL STORES.					
Arrow root,	lb.	10	5	3	
Candles (sperm),	lb.	2	1	1	
Farina,	lb.	10	5	3	
Ginger (fluid extract),	lb.	1	½	¼	
Nutmegs,	oz.	8	4	2	
Tea,	lb.	30	15	7	
Whisky, bottles of,	doz.	2	1	½	
BEDDING.					
Blankets, woolen,	no.	20–40	10–20	10	Brown.
Blanket cases,	no.	1 for	10 bla	nkets.	Of canvass, after pattern.
Gutta percha cloth,	yds.	8	4	2	
" " bed covers,	no.	8	4	2	So constructed as to form, when united, a continuous spread or covering.
Musquito bars,	no.	12	6	4	

FURNITURE AND DRESSINGS.

Bandages, roller, assorted,	doz.	14	7	4	
" suspensory, assorted,	no.	12	6	4	
Binders' boards,	no.	18	9	5	18 inches by 4.
Buckets, leather,	no.	4	2	2	BANDAGES.
Corks, assorted,	doz.	12	6	3	1 dozen, 1 inch wide, 1 yard long.
Corkscrews,	no.	2	1	1	2 " 2 " 3 "
Cotton batting,	lb.	2	1	½	2 " 2½ " 3 "
" wadding,	lb.	2	1	½	1 " 3 " 4 "
Flannel (red),	yds.	5	3	2	½ " 3½ " 5 "
Hatchets,	no.	2	1	1	½ " 4 " 6 "
Hones,	no.	1	1	1	4 inches by 1, in wood.
Ink, 2-ounce bottles,	no.	12	6	3	
Knapsack, hospital,	no.	—	—	—	According to pattern.
Lanterns,	no.	4	2	1	
Lint,	lb.	8	4	2	
Litters and stretchers, hand,	no.	—	—	—	} According to pattern.
" horse,	no.	—	—	—	}
Measures, graduated, assorted,	no.	4	2	2	6 oz., 2 oz., minim.
Medicine chests,	no.	—	—	—	
" cups and glasses,	no.	6	3	2	2 cups to 1 glass.
" panniers,	no.	—	—	—	
Mess chests,	no.	—	—	—	See note.
Mills, coffee,	no.	2	1	1	
Mortars and pestles, wedgewood,	no.	2	1	1	Small.
Muslin,	yds.	20	10	5	
Needles, sewing,	no.	25	25	25	Assorted, in a case.
Oiled silk or gutta percha tissue, or India rubber tissue,	yds.	8	4	2	
Pans, bed,	no.	2	1	1	Of hard India rubber or other material. Shovel.
Paper envelopes, assorted,	no.	100	50	25	50 letter, 25 note, 25 large. "Official Business" printed on each.
Paper, wrapping,	quires.	6	3	1	

TABLE FOR FIELD SERVICE—*Continued.*

ARTICLES.		QUANTITIES.			MEMORANDA.
		Reg't 3 mos.	Bat. 3 mos.	Com. 3 mos.	
FURNITURE AND DRESSINGS—*Continued.*					
Paper, writing,	quires.	12	6	3	2 foolscap, 6 letter, 4 note, white; blue ruled.
Pencils, hair,	no.	24	12	6	
" lead,	no.	12	6	3	
Pens, steel,	doz.	4	2	1	
Pill boxes (wood),	papers.	2	1	1	
" (tin),	no.	6	6	6	
Pins, assorted,	papers.	4	2	2	Large and medium.
Razors,	no.	1	1	1	
Razor strops,	no.	1	1	1	
Scales and weights, apothecary's,	sets.	1	1	1	
Scissors,	no.	4	2	2	
Sheep skins, dressed,	no.	4	2	1	
Silk, surgeons',	oz.	½	¼	¼	
Silk, green,	yds.	1	½	½	
Spatulas,	no.	6	3	2	
Sponge (washed),	lb.	1	½	¼	
Tape,	pieces.	4	2	1	
Thread, linen,	oz.	2	1	1	
Tiles,	no.	2	1	1	

Towels,	no.	40	20	10	
Twine,	lb.	½	¼	¼	
Urinals,	no.	4	2	1	
Vials, assorted,	doz.	4	2	1	1 oz. and 2 oz.
Wafers (½ ounce boxes),	no.	1	1	1	
Wax, sealing,	sticks.	2	1	1	

NOTE.—FURNITURE OF MESS CHEST.

8 Basins, tin.
2 Boxes, pepper and salt.
6 Cups, tin.
4 Canisters, (for tea, coffee, sugar, and butter).
2 Dippers and ladles.
1 Grater.
1 Gridiron.
1 Kettle, tea, iron.
12 Knives and forks.
6 Mugs, (Britannia. ½ pint.)
1 Pan, frying.
1 Pan, sauce.
8 Plates (6) and dishes, (2), tin.
1 Pot, iron.
2 Pots, coffee and tea, tin.
12 Spoons, iron, (table 6, and tea 2).
1 Tray, tin.
6 Tumblers, tin.

REQUISITION FOR MEDICAL AND HOSPITAL SUPPLIES.

STATION: PERIOD:

From *to*

COMMAND: *Officers,* ; *Enlisted Men,* ; *All others entitled to Medicines,* ; *Total,*

ARTICLES.		On hand.	Wanted.	ARTICLES.		On hand.	Wanted.
MEDICINES.				Ammoniæ carbonatis,	oz.		
				" muriatis,	lb.		
Acaciæ,	lb.			Anthemidis,	lb.		
Acidi acetici,	lb.			Antimoni et potass. tartratis,	oz.		
" arseniosi,	oz.			Argenti nitratis (crystals)	oz.		
" benzoici,	oz.			" " (fused)	oz.		
" citrici,	lb.			Arnicæ,	lb.		
" muriatici,	lb.			Assafœtidæ,	oz.		
" nitrici,	lb.			Bismuthi subnitratis,	oz.		
" sulphurici,	lb.			Camphoræ,	lb.		
" " aromatici,	lb.			Cardamomi,	oz.		
" tannici,	oz.			Catechu,	lb.		
" tartarici,	lb.			Ceræ albæ,	lb.		
Aetheris sulphurici loti,	lb.			Cerati resinæ,	lb.		
Alcoholis,	bott.			" simplicis,	lb.		
Aluminis,	lb.			" zinci carbonatis,	lb.		
Ammoniaci,	lb.			Chloroformi,	lb.		

Collodii,	oz.
Copaibæ,	lb.
Creasoti,	oz.
Cretæ preparatæ,	lb.
Cupri sulphatis,	oz.
Emplastri adhæsivi,	yds.
" cantharidis,	lb.
" ferri,	lb.
" hydrargyri,	lb.
" ichthyocollæ,	yds.
Extracti belladonnæ,	oz.
" buchu fluidi,	lb.
" colchici acetici,	oz.
" colocynthidis comp.,	oz.
" colombæ fluidi,	lb.
" conii,	oz.
" cubebæ fluidi,	lb.
" gentianæ fluidi,	lb.
" glycyrrhizæ,	lb.
" hyoscyami,	oz.
" ipecacuanhæ fluidi,	lb.
" piperis fluidi,	oz.
" pruni virg. fluidi,	lb.
" rhei fluidi,	lb.
" sarsaparillæ fluidi,	lb.
" senegæ fluidi,	lb.
" sennæ fluidi,	lb.
" taraxaci fluidi,	lb.
" valerianæ fluidi,	oz.
" zingiberis fluidi,	lb.
Ferro iodidi,	oz.
" et quiniæ citratis,	oz.
" sulphatis,	oz.
Gambogiæ,	oz.
Guaiaci resinæ,	lb.
Hydrargyri chloridi corr,,	oz.
" " mitis,	lb.
" cum creta,	lb.
" iodidi,	oz.
" oxidi rubri,	oz.
Iodinii,	oz.
Lini,	lb.
Liquoris ammoniæ,	lb.
" ferri iodidi,	lb.
" potass. arsenitis,	oz.
" sodæ chlorinatæ,	bott.
" zinci chloridi,	bott.
Magnesiæ,	lb.
" sulphatis,	lb.
Massæ pil. hydrargyri,	oz.
Mellis despumati,	lb.
Morphiæ sulphatis,	dr.
Myrrhæ,	lb.
Olei anisi,	oz.
" cajuputi,	oz.
" caryophylli,	oz.
" cinnamomi,	oz.
" menthæ piperitæ,	oz.
" morrhuæ,	bott.
" olivæ,	bott.
" origani,	oz.
" ricini,	qt. bott.
" terebinthinæ,	qt. bott.
" tiglii,	dr.
Opii,	lb.
Picis abietis,	lb.
Plumbi acetatis,	lb.
Potassæ acetatis,	lb.

Requisition for Medical and Hospital Supplies—*Continued.*

Articles.		On hand.	Wanted.	Articles.		On hand.	Wanted.
Potassæ bicarbonatis,	lb.			Quassiæ,	lb.		
" bitartratis,	lb.			Quiniæ sulphatis,	oz.		
" chloratis,	lb.			Rhei,	oz.		
" nitratis,	lb.			Sacchari,	lb.		
" sulphatis,	lb.			Saponis,	lb.		
Potassii cyanureti,	dr.			Scillæ,	oz.		
" iodidi,	oz.			Serpentariæ,	lb.		
Pruni virginianæ,	lb.			Sodæ bicarbonatis,	lb.		
Pulveris acaciæ,	lb.			" boratis,	lb.		
" aloes,	oz.			" et potass. tartratis,	lb.		
" cantharidis,	oz.			Spigeliæ,	lb.		
" capsici,	lb.			Spiritus ammon. aromatici,	oz.		
" cinchonæ,	lb.			" ætheris compositi,	lb.		
" ferri,	oz.			" " nitrici,	lb.		
" " per sulphatis,	oz.			" lavandulæ comp.,	lb.		
" glycyrrhizæ,	oz.			" vini gallici,	bott.		
" ipecacuanhæ,	lb.			Strychniæ,	dr.		
" " et opii,	lb.			Sulphuris loti,	lb.		
" jalapæ,	oz.			Syrupi scillæ,	lb.		
" lini,	lb.			Tincturæ aconiti radicis,	lb.		
" opii,	lb.			" digitalis,	oz.		
" rhei,	oz.			" ergotæ (Dublin)	oz.		
" sabinæ,	oz.			" ferri chloridii,	lb.		
" sinapis nigræ,	lb.			" veratri viridis,	oz.		
" ulmi,	lb.			Unguenti hydrargyri,	lb.		

Unguenti hydrargyri nitratis,	lb.
Veratriæ,	dr.
Vini colchici seminis,	lb.
Zinci acetatis,	oz.
" sulphatis,	oz.

12

INSTRUMENTS.

Buck's spongeholder for the throat,	no.
Cupping glasses or tins,	no.
Dissecting,	sets.
Lancets, spring,	no.
" thumb,	no.
Obstetrical,	sets.
Pocket,	sets.
Probangs,	no.
Pulleys,	sets.
Scarificators,	no.
Splints (assorted),	sets.
Stethoscopes,	no.
Stomach pump and case,	no.
Syringes, enema,	no.
" penis, glass,	no.
" " metallic,	no.
" vagina,	no.
Teeth extracting,	sets.
Tongue depressor (hinge),	no.
Tourniquets, field,	no.
" spiral,	no.
Trusses, hernia,	no.

BOOKS.

Anatomy,	cop.
Chemistry,	cop.
Dispensatory,	cop.
Medical dictionary,	cop.
" formulary,	cop.
" jurisprudence and toxicology,	cop.
" practice,	cop.
Obstetricy,	cop.
Regulations for medical department,	cop.
Surgery,	cop.
Blank,	no.
Case,	no.
Meteorological register,	no.
Order and letter,	no.
Prescription,	no.
Register,	no.
Requisitions, Returns, Reports of sick,	no.

HOSPITAL STORES.

Arrow root,	lb.
Barley,	lb.
Cinnamon,	lb.
Cloves,	oz.
Cocoa,	lb.
Farina,	lb.
Ginger, ground (Jamaica).	lb.
Nutmegs,	oz.
Tea,	lb.
Whisky, bottles of,	doz.
Wine, bottles of,	doz.

Requisition for Medical and Hospital Supplies—*Continued.*

Articles.		On hand.	Wanted.
BEDDING.			
Bed sacks,	no.		
Bedsteads, iron,	no.		
Blankets, woolen,	no.		
Coverlets,	no.		
Gutta percha cloth,	yds.		
Mattresses,	no.		
Musquito bars,	no.		
Pillow cases,	no.		
" ticks,	no.		
Sheets,	no.		
FURNITURE, DRESSINGS, Etc.			
Bandages, suspensory,	no.		
Binder's boards,	no.		
Corks, assorted,	doz.		
Cork screws,	no.		
Cotton batting,	lb.		
" wadding,	lb.		
Flannel, red,	yds.		
Funnels, glass,	no.		
" tin,	no.		
Hatchets,	no.		

Articles.		On hand.	Wanted.
Hones (in wood),	no.		
Ink powder,	papers.		
Inkstands,	no.		
Linen,	yds.		
Lint,	lb.		
Measures, graduated,	no.		
" tin,	sets.		
Medicine cups and glasses,	no.		
Mills, coffee,	no.		
Mortars and pestles, glass,	no.		
" " iron,	no.		
" " wedgewood,	no.		
Muslin,	yds.		
Needles, sewing,	no.		
Oiled silk, or gutta percha tissue, or India rubber tissue,	yds.		
Pans, bed,	no.		
Paper envelopes,	no.		
Paper, filtering,	quires.		
" wrapping,	quires.		
" writing,	quires.		
Pencils, hair,	no		
" lead,	no.		
Pens, steel,	doz.		
Pill boxes,	papers.		

Pill machine,	no.
Pins, assorted,	papers.
Quills,	no.
Rain gauges,	no.
Razors,	no.
Razor strops,	no.
Scales and weights, apothecary's,	sets.
" " shop,	sets.
Scissors,	no.
Sheep skins, dressed,	no.
Silk, surgeon's,	oz.
" green,	yds.
Spatulas,	no.
Sponge,	lb.
Tape,	pieces.
Thermometers and hygrometers,	no.
Thermometers,	no.
Thread, linen,	oz.
Tiles,	no.
Tow,	lb.
Towels,	no.
Twine,	lb.
Urinals,	no.
Vials, assorted,	doz.
Wafers (½ oz. boxes),	no.
Wax, sealing,	sticks.

ARTICLES FOR FIELD SERVICE ONLY.

Brominii,	oz.
Pilul. Cathartic. comp. (U. S.),	doz.
" opii (U. S.),	doz.
" quinæ sulphatis (3 grs.),	doz.
Tincturæ opii,	oz.
Syringes, penis (India rubber),	no.
Anatomy (surgical),	cop.
Surgery (operative),	cop.
Thompson's Conspectus,	cop.
Candles, sperm,	lbs.
Blanket cases,	no.
Gutta percha bed covers,	no.
Bandages, assorted,	doz.
Buckets, leather,	no.
Ink (2 oz. bottles),	no.
Knapsacks (hospital),	no.
Lanterns,	no.
Litters and stretchers (hand),	no.
" " (horse),	no.
Medicine chests,	no.
" panniers,	no.
Mess chests,	no.
Pill boxes (tin),	no.

....

Surgeon U. S. Army.

Date:

N. B.—Requisitions will exhibit the quantity of each article "on hand," whether more be wanted or not. They will be transmitted in duplicate, and by different mails.

FORM FOR REQUISITION FOR FORAGE.

REQUISITION *for Forage for* *Private Horses in the service of* *U. S. Army at* *for* *days, commencing the* *of* , 18 , *and ending the* *of* , 18 .

DATE.	Number of horses.	DAILY ALLOWANCE FOR EACH.				TOTAL ALLOWANCE.				REMARKS.
		CORN.	OATS.	HAY.	FODDER.	CORN.	OATS.	HAY.	FODDER.	
		Pounds.	Pounds.	Pounds.	Pounds.	Pounds.	Pounds.	Pounds.	Pounds.	
Total,	-	-	-	-	-					

I certify, on honor, that the above Requisition is correct and just, and that I have not drawn forage for any part of the time above charged.

....

RECEIVED at , the of , 18 , of Quartermaster U. S. Army, pounds of corn, pounds of oats, pounds of hay, pounds of fodder, in full of the above requisition.

[SIGNED IN DUPLICATE]

....

FORM FOR REQUISITION FOR STRAW.

Requisition for Straw, for the Hospital of the Regiment of commanded by , for the month of , 18 .

STATION.	Non-commissioned officers, musicians and privates.	Laundresses.	Servants.	Total drawn for.	Monthly allowance to each.	Total allowance.	REMARKS.
					Pounds.	Pounds.	
Total, - -							

I certify, on honor, that the above Requisition is correct and just, and that straw has not been drawn for any part of the time above charged.

....
Surgeon.

Received at , the of 18 , of Quartermaster United States Army, pounds of straw, in full of the above requisition.

(SIGNED DUPLICATES.)

....
Surgeon.

FORM FOR REQUISITION FOR FUEL.

Requisition for Fuel for the Hospital at *for the month of* 18 .

	WOOD.			COAL.		REMARKS.
	Cords.	Feet.	Inches.	Bushels.	Pounds.	
						No. of Fires.
Total, - - - -						

I certify on honor, that the above requisition is correct and just, and that I have not drawn fuel for any part of the time above charged.

RECEIVED at , the of , 18 , of , Quartermaster U. S. Army, cord feet inches of wood, of coal, in full of the above requisition.

(SIGNED IN DUPLICATE.)

FORM FOR ACCOUNTS OF PURCHASES.

The United States

1861. *To A. B.* *Dr.*

1861.		$	cts.
April.	For		

I certify that the above articles were purchased for the use of the Hospital at this post.

....

RECEIVED at of the sum of in full of the above account.

A. B.

PROVISION RETURN.

Provision Return for men in Hospital for   *days, commencing on the*   *, and ending on the*   18 .

STATION.	No. of days.	No. of men.	Total.	RATIONS OF Pork.	Beef.	Flour.	Rice or Beans.	Sugar.	Coffee.	Candles.	Soap.	Salt.	Vinegar.	REMARKS.
														Steward. Nurses. Sick. Total.
Due,														
Drawn,	-	-	-											
Retained,	-	-	-											

.... *Surgeon.*

RETURN OF HOSPITAL STORES, FURNITURE, ETC.

Return of Hospital Stores, Bedding, Furniture, Dressings, etc., received, expended, issued and
13 *remaining on hand at for the ending* 18 . .

ARTICLES.	On hand at last return.	Received since last return.	Total to be accounted for.	Expended with the sick.	Issued.	Lost or destroyed by unavoidable accident.	Worn out or unfit for use.	Total expended, issued, etc.	On hand.	REMARKS.
HOSPITAL STORES.										
Arrow root, - -										
Barley, - - -										
Etc., etc.										

RETURN OF MEDICINES, ETC.

Return of Medicines, Instruments, and Books, received, expended, Issued, and remaining on hand at for the ending 18 .

ARTICLES.	On hand at last return.	Received since last return.	Total to be accounted for.	Expended with the sick.	Issued.	Lost or destroyed by unavoidable accident.	Worn out or unfit for use.	Total expended, issued, etc.	On hand.	REMARKS.
MEDICINES.										
Acaciæ, - - - - lb.										
Acidi acetici, - - - lb.										
" arseniosi (arsenic), - oz.										
Etc., etc.										

REGISTER OF SICK.

No.	NAMES.	Rank.	Regiment.	Company.	Complaint.	Admitted.	For duty.	On furlough.	Deserted.	Discharged.	Died.	REMARKS.

PRESCRIPTION AND DIET BOOK.

NAMES.	April 1st.	2d.	3d.	4th.	5th.	6th.

MUSTER AND DESCRIPTIVE ROLL, ETC.

Muster and Descriptive Roll and Account of Pay and Clothing of

No.	NAMES.	RANK.	DESCRIPTION.						WHERE BORN.		OCCUPATION.	ENLISTED.				LAST PAID.		BOUNTY.		REMARKS.
			Age.	Eyes.	Hair.	Complexion.	Feet.	Inches.	State or kingdom.	Town or county.		When.	Where.	By whom.	Period.	By pay-master.	To what time.	$ Paid.	$ Due.	

CLOTHING ACCOUNT.

NAMES.	Wool Overalls.	Cotton Overalls.	Wool Jackets.	Cotton Jackets.	Cotton Shirts.	Flannel Shirts.	Boots.	Stockings.	Blankets.	Forage Caps.	Great Coats.	Great Coat straps.	Leather Stocks.	Drawers.					Date of issue.	BY WHOM ISSUED.

I certify that the above is a correct transcript from the Records of this Office.

....

SURGEON'S MORNING REPORT.

Morning Report of the Surgeon at ,

DATE.	Company.	REMAINING AT LAST REPORT.		Taken sick.	TOTAL.		Returned to duty.	Discharged.	Died.	REMAINING.		REMARKS.
		In Hospital.	In Quarters.		In Hospital.	In Quarters.				In Hospital.	In Quarters.	

DISCHARGES ON SURGEON'S CERTIFICATE, AND DEATHS.

NAME.		Rank.	Regiment.	Company.	Disease.	Date of discharge from service.	Date of death.
Surname.	Christian name.						

REMARKS.

NOTE.—Discharges on surgeon's certificate, and deaths occurring among those of the command *not* on sick report, will be also reported, but separated from the others by a double line drawn across the page. The remarks will in each case specify the manner in which the disease originated, when it is known.

REPORT OF SICK AND WOUNDED.

Report of the sick and wounded at *for the quarter ending* 18 .

CLASSES OF DISEASES.	TAKEN SICK OR RECEIVED INTO HOSPITAL DURING THE QUARTER.										
	Month, - - - -	FIRST.		SECOND.		THIRD.		TOTAL BY EACH DISEASE.		TOTAL BY EACH CLASS.	
	Specific diseases.	Cases.	Deaths.	Cases.	Deaths.	Cases.	Deaths.	Cases.	Deaths.	Cases.	Deaths.
Fevers.	Febris Congestiva, - - -										
	Febris Continua Communis, -										
	Febris Intermittens Quotidiana,										
	Febris Intermittens Tertiana,										
	Febris Intermittens Quartana, -										
	Febris Remittens, - - -										
	Febris Typhoides, - - -										
	Febris Typhus, - - -										
	Febris Typhus Icterodes, -										
	All other diseases of this class,										
Eruptive fevers.	Erysipelas, - - - -										
	Rubeola, - - - - -										
	Scarlatina, - - - -										
	Variola, - - - - -										
	Varioloides, - - - -										
	All other diseases of this class,										

Diseases of the organs connected with the digestive system.	Cholera Asiatica, - - -										
	Cholera Morbus, - - -										
	Colica, - - - - -										
	Constipatio, - - - -										
	Diarrhœa Acuta, - - -										
	Diarrhœa Chronica, - -										
	Dysenteria Acuta, - - -										
	Dysenteria Chronica, - -										
	Dyspepsia, - - - -										
	Enteritis, - - - -										
	Gastritis, - - - -										
	Hæmatemesis, - - -										
	Hepatitis Acuta, - - -										
	Hepatitis Chronica, - -										
	Icterus, - - - -										
	Parotitis, - - - -										
	Peritonitis, - - - -										
	Splenitis, - - - -										
	Tonsillitis, - - - -										
	All other diseases of this class,										
Diseases of the respiratory system.	Asthma, - - - - -										
	Bronchitis Acuta, - - -										
	Bronchitis Chronica, - -										
	Catarrhus Epidemicus, - -										
	Catarrhus, - - - -										
	Hæmoptysis, - - -										
	Laryngitis, - - - -										
	Phthisis Pulmonalis, - -										
	Pleuritis, - - - -										
	Pneumonia, - - - -										
	All other diseases of this class,										
Carry forward,											

REPORT OF SICK AND WOUNDED—*Continued.*

CLASSES OF DISEASES.	TAKEN SICK OR RECEIVED INTO THE HOSPITAL DURING THE QUARTER.										
	Month, - - - -	FIRST.		SECOND.		THIRD.		TOTAL BY EACH DISEASE.		TOTAL BY EACH CLASS.	
	Specific diseases.	Cases.	Deaths.	Cases.	Deaths.	Cases.	Deaths.	Cases.	Deaths.	Cases.	Deaths.
Diseases of the circulatory system.	Anæmia, - - - - -										
	Aneurisma, - - - -										
	Angina Pectoris, - - -										
	Carditis, - - - -										
	Endocarditis, - - - -										
	Pericarditis, - - -										
	Phlebitis, - - - -										
	Varicocele, - - - -										
	Varix, - - - - -										
	All other diseases of this class.										
Diseases of the brain and nervous system.	Apoplexia, - - - -										
	Cephalalgia, - - -										
	Cerebritis, - - - -										
	Chorea, - - - -										
	Delirium Tremens, - - -										
	Epilepsia, - - - -										
	Ictus Solis, - - - -										
	Irritatio Spinalis, - -										
	Mania, - - - - -										

	Melancholia, - - -										
	Meningitis, - - - -										
	Neuralgia, - - - -										
	Paralysis, - - - -										
	Tetanus, - - - -										
	All other diseases of this class,										
Diseases of the urinary and genital organs, and venereal affections.	Bubo Syphiliticum, - -										
	Calculus, - - - -										
	Cystitis, - - - - -										
	Diabetes, - - - -										
	Enuresis, - - - -										
	Gonorrhœa, - - - -										
	Ischuria et Dysuria, - -										
	Nephritis, - - - -										
	Orchitis, - - - - -										
	Sarcocele, - - - -										
	Strictura Urethræ, - - -										
	Syphilis Primitiva, - -										
	Syphilis Consecutiva, - -										
	Ulcus Penis Non Syphiliticum,										
	All other diseases of this class,										
Diseases of the serous exhalent vessels.	Anasarca, - - - -										
	Ascites, - - - -										
	Hydrarthrus, - - - -										
	Hydrocele, - - - -										
	Hydrothorax, - - - -										
	All other diseases of this class,										
Diseases of the fibrous & muscular structures	Lumbago, - - - -										
	Podagra, - - - -										
	Rheumatismus Acutus, - -										
	Rheumatismus Chronicus, -										
	All other diseases of this class,										
Carry forward,											

REPORT OF SICK AND WOUNDED—*Continued.*

CLASSES OF DISEASES.	TAKEN SICK OR RECEIVED INTO THE HOSPITAL DURING THE QUARTER. Month, - - - -	FIRST.		SECOND.		THIRD.		TOTAL BY EACH DISEASE.		TOTAL BY EACH CLASS.	
	Specific diseases.	Cases.	Deaths.	Cases.	Deaths.	Cases.	Deaths.	Cases.	Deaths.	Cases.	Deaths.
Abscesses and ulcers.	Abscessus, - - - -										
	Anthrax, - - - -										
	Fistula, - - - - -										
	Paronychia, - - - -										
	Phlegmon, - - - -										
	Ulcus, - - - - -										
	All other diseases of this class,										
Wounds and injuries.	Ambustio, - - - -										
	Concussio Cerebri, - -										
	Compressio Cerebri, - -										
	Contusio, - - - -										
	Fractura, - - - -										
	Gelatio, - - - -										
	Hernia, - - - - -										
	Luxatio, - - - -										
	Morsus Serpentis, - - -										
	Punitio, - - - -										
	Sub-luxatio, - - - -										
	Vulnus Incisum, - - -										

	Vulnus Contusum vel Laceratum,										
	Vulnus Punctum, - - -										
	Vulnus Sclopeticum, - -										
	All other diseases of this class,										
Diseases of the eye.	Amaurosis, - - - -										
	Cataracta, - - - -										
	Hemeralopia, - - - -										
	Iritis, - - - - -										
	Nyctalopia, - - - -										
	Ophthalmia, - - -										
	Retinitis, - - - -										
	All other diseases of this class,										
Diseases of the ear.	Otalgia, - - - - -										
	Otitis, - - - - -										
	Otorrhœa, - - - -										
	Surditas, - - - -										
	All other diseases of this class,										
All other diseases.	Anchylosis, - - - -										
	Atrophia, - - -										
	Bubo Simplex, - - -										
	Cachexia, - - - -										
	Debilitas, - - - -										
	Ebrietas, - - - -										
	Epistaxis, - - - -										
	Exostosis, - - - -										
	Hæmorrhois, - - - -										
	Hæmatocele, - - -										
	Morbi Cutis, - - - -										
	Necrosis, - - - -										
	Nostalgia, - - - -										
	Odontalgia, - - - -										
Carry forward,											

REPORT OF SICK AND WOUNDED—*Continued.*

CLASSES OF DISEASES.	TAKEN SICK OR RECEIVED INTO THE HOSPITAL DURING THE QUARTER.										
	Month, - - - -	FIRST.		SECOND.		THIRD.		TOTAL BY EACH DISEASE.		TOTAL BY EACH CLASS.	
	Specific diseases.	Cases.	Deaths.	Cases.	Deaths.	Cases.	Deaths.	Cases.	Deaths.	Cases.	Deaths.
All other diseases.	Prolapsus Ani, - - -										
	Scirrhus, - - - -										
	Scrobutus, - - - -										
	Scrofula, - - - -										
	Suicidium, - - - -										
	Toxicum, - - - -										
	Tumores, - - - -										
	Vermes, - - - -										
	Morbi Varii, - - - -										
	Total, - - - -										

Report of Sick and Wounded—*Continued.*

GENERAL SUMMARY.

REMAINING LAST REPORT.			Taken sick during the quarter.	Aggregate.	Sent to general hospital.	Returned to duty.	On furlough.	Discharged.	Deserted.	Died.	REMAIN-ING.			MEAN STRENGTH.				Number treated.	Deaths.	Ratio per 1,000 of mean strength.	
Sick.	Convalescent.	Total.									Sick.	Convalescent.	Total.	Months.	Officers.	Enlisted men.	Total.			Cases.	Deaths.
														Total.							
														Ratio per qr.							

DIRECTIONS.

In regard to this Report, the utmost punctuality and exactness will be required. It will be accompanied with a general Sanitary Report, to be written on alternate pages of foolscap paper, with a margin of one inch on the left side of each page, and to be folded in four equal folds; in which the medical officer will furnish information respecting all those agencies which may have influenced the sickness and mortality of the troops—such as the medical topography of the station; the climate; prevalent diseases in the vicinity; the duty and employment of the troops; the nature of their barrack and hospital accommodations; diet; water; clothing, and general habits of the men as to cleanliness, temperance, etc. Cases of unusual interest will be reported in detail. Diseases of women and children, if given, must be reported separately. No duplicate of this report is required.

MUSTER

Muster Roll of Steward, Wardmaster, Cooks, Nurses and Matrons,
the day of , 18 , when last

No.	NAMES. Present and absent.	HOW MUSTERED IN THE ARMY.						
		Rank.	Company.	Regiment.	ENLISTED.			
					When.	Where.	By whom.	Period.

RECAPITULATION.			Steward.	Wardmaster.	Cooks.	Nurses.	Matrons.	Total.	Total last month.
PRESENT. - -		For duty, - - - - -							
		Sick, - - - - -							
		In arrest, or confinement, -							
ABSENT. - -		On detached service, -							
		On furlough, - - -							
		Without leave, - -							
		Sick, - - - - -							
		In arrest, or confinement,							
STRENGTH—Present and Absent, - - -									
Alterations since last Muster.	Joined. -	Enlisted in hospital, -							
		By re-enlistment, - -							
		By transfer, - - -							
		From desertion, - - -							
	Discharged.	Expiration of service, -							
		For disability, - - -							
		By sentence of G. C. Martial,							
		By civil authority, - -							
		By order, - - -							
		Transferred, - - -							
	Died. - -	Killed in action, - -							
		Of wounds, - - -							
		From disease, etc., - -							
		Deserted, - - - -							

ROLL.

attached to the Hospital of , army of the United States, from mustered, to the day of , 18 .

ATTACHED TO HOSPITAL.		LAST PAID. (See note 7 of Remarks.)		BOUNTY. Act June 17, '50. (See note 4 of Remarks.)		NAMES.	REMARKS.
When.	How employed.	By paymaster.	To what time.	Paid. Dolls.	Due. Dolls.	Present.	

I certify, on honor, that this Muster Roll is made out in the manner required by the printed notes; that it exhibits the true state of the Hospital Department for the period herein mentioned; that the "Remarks" set opposite each name are accurate and just; and that the "Recapitulation" exhibits in every particular the true state of the Hospital, as required by the Regulations and the Rules and Articles of War.

STATION:

DATE:

....

Surgeon, in charge of Hospital.

I certify, on honor, that I have carefully examined this Muster Roll; that I have mustered and minutely inspected the hospital attendants; and that the police and general condition of the Hospital Department is found to be as follows.

....

Inspector and Mustering Officer.

MUSTER ROLL—*Continued.*

NOTES.

1.—Under the head of REMARKS, the *date* of any soldier's *joining*, whether *originally*, or from *any absence;* all changes of rank, by *promotion, appointment*, or *reduction*, with *date* of same, and *No., date*, etc., of order; all *authorized stoppages, fines, sentences*, with *No., date*, etc., of order, etc.; in case of ABSENCE, the *nature* and *commencement* of, *No., date*, etc., of order, and *period* assigned for same (to be *repeated on every roll while it lasts*); if *wounded* in battle, or *injured on duty*—if *sick*, or *confined*, a remark to that effect, etc., must be *carefully stated* opposite to the name of the person concerned, *with everything else necessary, either to account fully for every individual, to guide the paymaster, or ensure justice to the soldier, and to the United States.*

2.—In noting STOPPAGES to be made for *loss* or *damage* to public property, the *gross amount* due for *Ordnance, Horse Equipments, Clothing, etc.*, will be *separately* stated in the order enumerated in par. 1187, G. R.

3.—Additional pay, due under Sec. 2, Act of Aug. 4, 1854, will be thus noted, viz.: "For 1st re-enlist., $2 pr. mo.;" or, "For 2d re-enlist., $3 pr. mo.;" or, "For 3d re-enlist., $4 pr. mo.;" etc. That due under Sec. 3 of the same act, thus: "For cert. of merit, $2 per mo." That due under Sec. 4 of the same act, thus: "In lieu of comm., $2 pr. mo."

4.—The *installments* of Bounty due under Sec. 3, Act of June 17, 1850, are paid as follows: $\frac{1}{10}$, $\frac{1}{8}$, $\frac{1}{6}$, $\frac{1}{4}$, at the end of the 1st, 2d, 3d, and 4th years, respectively, the remainder at the expiration of enlistment; and will, under the head of REMARKS, be noted thus: "Ret'd Bounty due, 1st (or 2d, 3d, etc.) inst. $—." See G. O. 20 of 1850. *Besides* which, in the columns headed "BOUNTY PAID" and "BOUNTY DUE," must be entered in figures, the *whole amount hitherto paid*, and the *whole amount yet due*, on account of said bounty.

5.—The "three months' extra pay," for re-enlistment, under Sec. 29, Act of July 5, 1838, being paid by the recruiting officer, should not be noted on the muster rolls.

6.—The roll of those *belonging to the hospital*, will be immediately followed by that of those who, since last muster, *have ceased to belong to it.* These will be classed in the following order, viz.: *Discharged, Transferred, Died, Deserted;* and the *utmost particularity* will be observed in the *remarks* concerning them. *Date* and *place* will, *in every case*, be given; and *No., date*, etc., of *orders*, or *description of authority*, be always carefully specified. Soldiers discharged *and re-enlisted*, or who have deserted *and been retaken*, since last muster, have their place in *both* of the above rolls.

7.—The remark "*discharge and final statements given*" will be made opposite to the name of every discharged soldier, to whom such papers *have actually been given*. But the blank spaces under the head of Last Paid, are to be filled as usual.

8.—In all cases of "*re-enlistment*" prior to the expiration of the term of service, the *discharge* on the old enlistment will be given at the time the soldier "re-enlists," from and on which day, his pay on the *new* enlistment will commence.

9.—Within *three* days after each regular muster, the mustering officer or commandant of the post, will transmit to the Adjutant General a copy of the *muster roll* of each company. Blanks will be supplied from the Adjutant General's Office, and will be *acknowledged* on the first muster roll forwarded after their receipt.

RECORD

Of Events which may be necessary or useful for future reference of the War Department, or for present information.

PAY ROLL OF THE HOSPITAL.

Pay Roll of the Hospital, from the day of , 18 , when last paid, to the day of , 18

Period paid for.		Pay per month.	Amount of pay.		Retained pay.		Bounty.		Total am't due.		Am't of stoppages.		Balance. paid.		Received payment of.	Witness.
Months.	Days.	Dolls.	Dolls.	Cts.	Dolls.	Cts.	Paid. Dolls.	Due. Dolls.	Dolls.	Cts.	Dolls.	Cts.	Dolls.	Cts.		

NOTE.—Three muster and pay rolls are made at each muster—one to be retained with the hospital records, and two for the Paymaster. One *muster* roll is at the same time forwarded to the Adjutant General. The muster and pay roll blank is used for this purpose, the "pay roll" portion being cut off. See "General Orders," No. 9, of February 12 1851.

Norman Publishing is a division of Jeremy Norman & Company, Inc., leading international dealers in rare books and manuscripts in the history of medicine and science.

The following people collaborated on the production of *Hand-Book for the Military Surgeon:*

Diana Hook, Associate Editor
Steven Hiatt, Copy Editor
Jill Rotenberg, Project Manager
Martha Steele, Editorial Assistant
Seventeenth Street Studios, Designer

The layout was done by Donna Kelley at Zetatype Desktop Publishers of San Francisco, using Ventura Publisher. The type is Bodoni, a Postscript font from Adobe Systems.

Linotronic output by Pinnacle Type, San Francisco.

Printed and bound by Braun-Brumfield, Inc., Ann Arbor.

With its geometrical framework, the Norman Publishing logo resembles the constructed letters of the Renaissance, but there the resemblance ends. The logo incorporates the capital letter N within an arc of the logarithmic spiral, one of the most beautiful mathematical curves appearing in nature. It links together the graphic arts and the sciences, reflecting the dual commitments of Norman Publishing.

NORMAN
PUBLISHING ™